# YOUR BODY HEALS ITSELF

# YOUR BODY HEALS ITSELF

Richard Price

JUPITER : LONDON

First published in 1979 by
JUPITER BOOKS (LONDON) LIMITED

167 Hermitage Road, London N4 1LZ.



ISBN 0 906379 10 5

Composed on the Linotype-Paul VIP in 12-point Bembo and printed and bound in Great Britain by Tonbridge Printers Limited at their Peach Hall Works, Tonbridge, Kent.

# ACKNOWLEDGEMENTS

I AM INDEBTED to Dr. Joan Gomez and the Centaur Press Limited for the extracts from her *Dictionary of Symptoms;* to John Murray (Publishers) Limited for the use of extracts from J. Ellis Barker's *Cancer: How it is caused, How it can be prevented;* and to Neville Spearman Limited for quoting from *Food is Your Best Medicine!* by Henry G. Beiler MD.

*Richard Price*
Brighton, 1979.

# CONTENTS

# YOUR BODY HEALS ITSELF

*Chapter 1*

# THE NATURE-CURE APPROACH

THE FIRST TASK of individuals seeking good health is to adjust themselves to the laws of nature. To regard their bodies as a living organism, composed of cells whose function depends entirely on nutrition. The word 'nutrition' is used here to include oxygen, water and the circulation of the blood. Also they must obey the inexorable laws governing the health of the body, the breaking of which inevitably brings retaliation—mental and physical sickness.

Even if we ignore physical injuries, the body is a self-repairing organism, given a carefully balanced diet and a natural environment. However, there remains a nucleus of major ailments where self-treatment would be wrong and indeed dangerous. Medical diagnosis should *never* be attempted by unqualified persons. That is the responsibility and prerogative of a doctor; he alone has the equipment and ability to perform that important function.

Nature-cure methods emphasize the correct diet for a particular disorder and the appropriate vitamins and mineral supplements beneficial for each ailment, rather than indiscriminate swallowing of vitamin tablets daily, which may or may not be suitable for their specific disorder. This book will help sufferers derive the maximum benefit from using certain remedies. It is written without prejudice, favouritism, or any implied criticism of the medical profession. It is not intended as a 'cure-all' for disease, nor as an alternative to consulting a general practitioner. It is important that anyone experiencing a pain they do not understand, or cannot identify, should at once consult a doctor. Our intention is to endeavour to prevent certain common ailments; to examine their causes and symptoms with a view to self-treatment along nature-cure lines, provided they are not already being treated by a doctor or an osteopath.

Our purpose is to help sufferers to decide when to consult a physician, and when the ailment does not warrant troubling a busy doctor. We are concerned with symptoms rather than disease, as indicated by the chapter-headings. This book was suggested by one of my grateful customers, and I agreed to his request that these remedies should be recorded for the benefit of mankind.

He had been treated for rheumatism in his right arm and shoulder for years without success. Yet a simple remedy, costing only a few pence, relieved the pain and reduced the swelling in three weeks! This remedy is stated in full detail in Chapter 2. The list of remedies that follow may not always be successful in every case—75% would be a fair estimate. There are a wide variety of causes and many unknown factors involved, especially among elderly persons.

These simple remedies are offered in all sincerity, however ludicrous they appear at first glance. There is only one criterion — are they effective? They are quite harmless, mostly inexpensive, and some possess other virtues than those claimed by their manufacturers. Although the majority are nature-cure remedies, I have included a limited number of others because they are remarkably effective.

We are punished by our sins, not for them. This is especially true with regard to wrong eating, wrong living, drug addiction and excessive smoking. All kinds of diseases are of our own making, are mostly preventable, and can be remedied largely by our own hands. Immunity to pain cannot be obtained with money, only with correct nutrition, the right mental and moral attitude and self-discipline.

It is astonishing how frequently a simple natural remedy will prove effective, after a variety of orthodox treatments haved failed dismally. Nature heals in her own mysterious and inimitable manner. Man can only gaze in awe and wonder! The choice is, to use drugs having known and unknown harmful side-effects, or, safe natural remedies that work towards the elimination of disease.

These simple medicines have been selected solely for their therapeutic value from the wide range available in health shops. There is no intentional advertising and no manufacturer had any previous knowledge of my recommendations. Some of these remedies are of gipsy origin as Romany folk living close to nature share many of her secrets. Others are herbal preparations, and herbs have been used successfully for treating disease since the dawn of history. Doctors use nearly 200 herbs in their medicines today, while herbalists use over 300.

The value of herbal treatment is illustrated by the following anecdote. An English doctor on holiday in Africa was bitten by a venomous mamba snake, which normally means death in thirty minutes. He collapsed and his native bearer ran for the local witch-doctor. That worthy man calmly gathered a few herbs and placed them on the wound. The doctor recovered, but he never discovered the secret of those herbs!

It is plain common-sense to prevent disease by adopting personal health measures, rather than worrying about which are important, and which are trivial symptoms. Let us take a closer look at those remedies that work in harmony with nature. The chemicals for the restoration of health are provided by nature. Man cannot copy them successfully, but the search goes on.

I do not guarantee permanent cures, neither does orthodox treatment, with all the weight of medical science behind it. I do suggest they merit a fair trial, especially as they are harmless and non-addictive. They are presented in ordinary laymen's language, no Latin phrases—so dear to the heart of professional writers.

*Chapter 2*

# SYMPTOMS OF RHEUMATISM AND ARTHRITIS

IT IS ESTIMATED that half the population of this country suffer from rheumatism or arthritis in one form or another. Medical science continues to spend large sums searching for the 'wonder drug', but the disease steadily increases, while natural remedies are ignored or regarded with mistrust and suspicion. Yet gipsies do *not* suffer from rheumatic ailments and live happily to a ripe old age. Is it their untreated whole foods that give them immunity? Or, their ability to utilize nature's plentiful supply of herbs?

Perhaps an unbiased appraisal of some of the common causes of rheumatic ailments will provide the answer. And, I trust, will help sufferers who are very familiar with that depressing message 'you have to live with it'. The majority of patients swallow pills with apparent enjoyment, but only a minority are willing to adapt their meals to a strict healthy diet—the essential feature of nature-cure treatment. Medicine and diet functioning in harmony to bring about the desired result.

Sometimes drugs afford present relief and the patient appears to recover as a result of their use. This happens because nature has reserves of vital force to expel the poison and correct conditions caused by the ailment. The effect of the poison seems to be overcome for the time being as the patient feels more comfortable and the swelling has been reduced. But because his system is saturated with toxic poisons, the pain is bound to return sooner or later, and he is back to his former condition, or worse.

That familiar routine illustrates the importance of correct nutrition: nature's method of eliminating excess acid and toxins from the system. To break the habit of a lifetime is not easy. However, it is usually the main obstacle along the road to good health. Rheumatism is sometimes allied to, or part of another deep-seated ailment and only a doctor or an osteopath can make the necessary tests. Stiffness of joints is the nagging feature of rheumatic ailments, and anything that helps freer motion is beneficial, especially moist heat, hot baths and hot-water bottles.

Formerly, rheumatism was recognized as painful movements in muscles and ligaments, but of recent years it has become a 'blanket' ailment, covering almost any limitation of movement. This applies particularly to elderly persons who have been living on a diet over-weighted with protein and animal fat over the years. Rheumatism is not usually hereditary, except in so far as families continue the same diet and environment, and inevitably each generation suffers from the same diseases. Heredity is the popular excuse for complacency—until the pain becomes intense.

Rheumatic ailments can have a psychosomatic

origin—the pain is real, but the cause lies in an unsettled upheaval in the past. These cases need psychotherapy and there are competent practitioners who advertise their services in the health magazines. The psychological factor should not be overlooked, especially where physical treatment has failed to gain any response, or only partially succeeded. Practitioners will diagnose to what extent emotional stress has contributed to the cause of the disease.

Two popular items on the menu that are often consumed at the same time are alcohol and fats; these are liable to cause rheumatic conditions. Alcohol is assimilated into the system quickly and fat, formerly left in the body remains passive while the alcohol is digested. Fat is a source of energy provided it can be absorbed into the system. But in excess of the body's requirements it is stored in the tissues under the skin. The danger lies in the fact that there is no limit to the amount the body can store. The general process of digestion is completed in approximately five to six hours.

Certain fatty foods, e.g. roast pork, need four to five hours to digest owing to their fatty composition. Before they are completely digested, more food is poured into the over-worked stomach, and fat, or what are now fatty acids, begin to build up in the system. The body assimilates vegetable poly-unsaturated fats quickly and turns them into energy. Animal fat is a slower process and the stomach reacts in nature's inimitable way—excess acid returns to the blood stream instead of the waste channel. Verily *the* common cause of disease is food habits.

Eskimos stand in freezing cold water to build their salmon dams. Hindus, sailors, boilermen and many others perform hard physical tasks in very high temperatures. None of them suffer any ill-effects from these extremes of heat and cold; however, ingesting the wrong foods over a prolonged period is attacking the body from within, and that the body does *not* tolerate. Sickness is not the inevitable lot of mankind. It is nature hitting back when she receives the wrong fuel for her pre-ordained purpose.

Another cause of arthritis is muscular imbalance. It causes an artificial strain on the spine, e.g. poor posture, excessive use of certain muscles on one side of the body, such as ironing, carrying heavy shopping bags, playing tennis, etc. This condition needs *corrective* exercises under medical supervision, especially if there is a tendency towards arthrosis of the hip, or spinal arthritis. It's an elementary principle of physics—only muscles in balance function smoothly. Muscle imbalance affects persons of all ages and if not promptly corrected spreads right through the body.

An insidious cause of rheumatism is induced by the stomach losing an increasing amount of hydrochloric acid as people get on in years, with the result that proteins tend to pass through the body only partially digested. To counteract this food deficiency, the body is obliged to draw protein from the tissues, or from the muscles, causing rheumatism, or sometimes from the joints, causing arthritis. The obvious remedy is to make sure of adequate protein in the daily diet.

Rising sales figures of pre-packed medicines indicate

that more and more people are turning to self-medication. A wasteful practice if those medicines merely induce a false sense of well-being, having only marginal therapeutic value. The market is flooded with 'wonder cures', yet degenerative disease continues its upward march with its incalculable suffering to mankind. So much for their drugs! The human tragedy is that we have lost sight of, or have refused to recognize the recuperative power of the human body.

In medical language rheumatism is a general term applied to a wide range of degenerate affections of muscles and joints, and any superficial pain that defies prompt diagnosis. Sciatica, neuralgia, gout, lumbago, osteo-arthritis, are separate groups of rheumatism. As the following nature-cure remedies apply to every group, it is unnecessary to enumerate their specific symptoms here.

These remedies are not in any therapeutic order of merit, nor do they guarantee to prove beneficial in *every* case. They have been selected from a wide range, and are considered in general terms to have proved satisfactory. They are safe alternative remedies to drugs, perfectly harmless and with no side-effects. Here I have included a simple remedy especially recommended for the extremities. It costs about 20p at the greengrocers.

Cut a large onion in half and extract the juice by using a lemon-squeezer, or a garlic-crusher, which is used in a similar way to nutcrackers. Soak a pad of cotton-wool in the juice and apply to the affected parts every evening on retiring. It is important to rub well in until the juice has evaporated. Extracting the juice is a tedious business. It would be a sound investment for a group of sufferers to share an electric juicer, available in health shops.

Another remedy is wheat germ oil applied similarly to the above, and in addition, two tablespoons to be taken daily with meals. Olbas Oil (from health shops) relieves rheumatic pain and full directions are enclosed in every packet. Biochemic Tissue Salt Nat.Phos.No.10 is also a useful remedy. It neutralizes excess acid in the system and assists in its elimination. Garlic capsules, celery tablets and kelp tablets are all helpful for rheumatism, but are not always effective for every individual. For the relief of gout, rub into the toe pure turpentine; also, practise total abstinence from wine, acid juices, spirits and red meat.

Grandma's Remedy for the relief of rheumatic pain: 4 oz. camphorated oil, one teaspoonful of ammonia. The mixture to be applied externally to the affected parts. Crude black molasses is a popular remedy for rheumatism and certain other ailments. It tends to create an alkaline reaction that benefits sufferers. It is a natural evacuent, rich in potassium (the nerve nutrient) and also contains calcium and iron. Being very pungent it is best taken dissolved in hot water after meals.

Vegetex is another herbal tablet with a high alkaline content that neutralizes the acidity in the body and assists its passage through the system. It is not a laxative or a purgative. However, it tends to alleviate the pain and helps tired muscles regain their elasticity.

A gipsy remedy: gather fresh hydrangea leaves and slowly dry them out. Pour hot water on them and infuse for twelve hours. Strain off the liquid and take half a wine-glassful after meals.

The latest remedy is Devil's Claw tablets, which are advertised as having an immediate effect on rheumatism and arthritis. Free leaflets are available giving detailed information on the exceptional healing power of this bitter African herb, (priced at £2.17 for 84 tablets at the time of writing). Also, Calcium Pantothenic tablets help relieve arthritic sufferers when there is a deficiency of this vitamin in the system. Vitamin B complex tablets facilitate several bodily functions and they contain pantothenic acid.

Another little-known remedy is Minalka. A mineral compound from Denmark that has achieved 72% success in relieving rheumatic and arthritic pain. It counteracts the shortage of minerals in the popular diet and restores the natural balance of carbohydrates, fats and proteins. It is well worth three months trial. My final remedy is Bio-strath Rheumatic Elixir No. 5. Basically a yeast extract, it contains an extensive list of herbs, plus various minerals and nature's vital substances in concentrated form.

Linseed relieves arthritic pain in persons of all ages. An economical remedy it can be obtained for only 10p per ounce, or, the compost grown variety is available in packets at a higher price. Place a teaspoonful in a tea-strainer and pour hot water over it to wash out any dust. Eat a spoonful twice a day, reducing to once a day when the pain has gone.

The late Dr. Lincoln Williams relates an astonishing incident in his book, *To Each His Memories*. He suffered an acute attack of lumbago while on holiday in France. A friend suggested he called on a local fisherman for treatment. Although the doctor thought Nicolas the fisherman was a phoney, he agreed to go on condition that Nicolas was not aware that his patient was a doctor. On arrival at the cottage Nicolas requested the doctor to strip down to the waist and sit down. Then, going behind the doctor, Nicolas proceeded to massage the back of his neck. Dr. Williams promptly reminded him the pain was in the region of the lower back. Nicolas's reply surprised the worthy doctor. He said, 'Today is Wednesday, by Friday you will be quite free from pain.' To the doctor's amazement this actually happened!

A homely demonstration of the healing power within the human body. Nicolas released that power by touch, and taut nerves and tense muscles were immediately relaxed. Mother Nature, given the opportunity, does her work wisely and efficiently. To respond to her unwritten laws is the first step towards buoyant good health. Contrary to academic opinion—'you *don't* have to live with it'!

To obtain maximum results, the following diet should be used in conjunction with the aforementioned remedies:

100% wholemeal bread; vegetable margarine; fresh salads using lemon juice; fruit; cheese; eggs; milk; dates; figs; raisins; vegetable juices; green or root vegetables; fish, boiled preferably; raw sugar.

Avoid:

salt; white sugar; fried foods; ham and pork fat; chocolate and products containing chocolate; animal fats; rich mixtures; vinegar; salad cream; fatty and starchy foods; butter and butter products; plums; gooseberries; rhubarb.

*Chapter 3*

# HEALTH FOODS—THEIR RELATION TO SLIMMING

EATING HEALTH FOODS to build up the body, and slimming in order to reduce weight, is apparently a contradiction in terms. However, both affect the health and well-being of our physical bodies, therefore it is appropriate to present both facets of this diverse subject. In this connection there are five pertinent questions posed frequently in health shops. With slight variations they are as follows:

*Question*

Are health foods necessary ,to maintain good health?

*Answer*

They are definitely necessary to maintain good health, to relieve mental stress and the physical strain of modern living. Also, to fortify the body against disease and degeneration. Health foods are free from preservatives, cyclamates, artificial substances and adventitious additives of any description. These are some of the substances that can be lawfully added to foods: aldrin; anti-oxidants; emulsifiers; antibiotics; preservatives; nitrogen-trichloride; clorine-dioxide; etc. The chemicals used in the preparation of foods are not harmful in small doses, but the cumulative effect over a period of time is a matter for grave concern.

*Question*

Why are health foods dearer than other shop foods?

*Answer*

The term 'expensive' is purely relative when comparing the nutritional value of food. There is no commercial valuation of the joy and happiness of buoyant, glowing good health. Health foods do not contain any 'filling' to make up the weight, or prolong shelf life. For instance, the difference in price of health food jam made with raw sugar and the factory product is very small. Many factory jams are packed in 12 oz. jars. Health food jams are packed in 16 oz. jars, therefore the actual difference in value is infinitesimal. Imported mixtures of muisli are inevitably dearer than corn flakes, but mixed with corn flakes they add concentrated protein and flavour to the meal. Also one can make an economical muisli by using Muisli Base and wheat flakes. These are a whole wheat product flavoured with brown sugar and natural sea salt. For a delicious breakfast add raisins, barley kernels, grated apple, chopped dates, sultanas, and ground almonds. The extra cost of health foods to the average family would be approximately 40 to 50 pence per week. Measured in terms of good health, it is *very good* value for money.

*Question*

Will health foods help me to slim?

*Answer*

Health foods are designed to provide optimum good health, not to assist or encourage the reduction of body weight. They contain the equal or more in calories, weight for weight of competitive foods. However, if consumed with slimming tablets or a slimming regimen, they will help slimming in harmony with the natural laws of nutrition. It is important to adopt a balanced health food diet, accompanied by adequate exercise. This would tend to make you lose weight without the aid of slimming tablets.

*Question*

Which are the best slimming tablets?

*Answer*

The most effective and safest slimming tablets are the Minima brand, manufactured in Sweden and imported by Modern Health Products Limited. These do not need a special diet, but it is essential to follow the enclosed directions. This applies also to Hofels Reducing Plan Formula S, a reducing course available in health stores. The pack contains a specially controlled programme which slims the figure and contributes towards good health.

*Question*

Are slimming tablets effective without health foods?

*Answer*

Undoubtedly herbal slimming tablets are effective without health foods. However, their effectiveness is reduced if anyone is taking medicines which contain drugs, barbiturates, or artificial stimulants. The straight choice is in drugs or nature-cure remedies. They do not function happily together in the human body. That is a common pitfall that surrounds self-medication. Nature-cure remedies work best in harmony with nature and the natural principles inherent in all living things.

At this point I would like to correct some common misconceptions concerning slimming and its threat to health. Firstly, four or five pounds overweight does not warrant a strict course of dieting. The body weight naturally varies that amount according to one's environment, individual bone structure, or hereditary factors. Secondly, there is no such substance as a 'reducing food'. All food is subject to calorific content and nourishment demands calories.

Furthermore, dry toast, crispbreads, or cracker biscuits, spread with butter will *not* help to reduce weight. In fact butter is the slimmer's worst enemy. Also, it is dangerous to lose weight too quickly. The side-effects are irritability and stress caused by the strain on the nervous system. Because jockeys 'dry out' before a race to keep their weight down, the fallacy has spread that abstinence from liquids will automatically lose body weight. It might lose a few ounces, but the body's condition would re-adjust the shortage in two days. Moreover, it is dangerous to experiment with the balance of liquid in the body. Strict dieting and a shortage of water tends to cause constipation; therefore the second condition is worse than the first. In that event, use one of the remedies suggested in Chapter Four, and cancel the diet until the constipation has been alleviated.

Safe slimming involves reducing the calorific content of one's diet at the same time as increasing one's physical activities. Calories must be burned up by more exercise or the body continues to store up surplus fat. The danger lies in the fact that there is no limit to the amount the body can store.

Proteins stimulate the body to burn faster, while carbohydrates are the least desirable to the slimmer. A reasonable safety margin is a weight loss of two pounds a week. It is helpful to cut out butter and reduce animal fats to the minimum. Instead of butter use vegetable margarines made from sun-flower seed oil, Sun-o-life or similar brands. These cost about 3p more than butter, but we are buying to build health, not to satisfy hunger. These margarines contain stabilized wheat germ oil, plus vitamins A and D.

The calorie chart shows that one gramme of protein produces four calories, therefore, fats must be reduced for successful slimming and carbohydrates balanced on the four calorie basis. The daily menu should contain protein, fats and carbohydrates, but reduce the size of the portions. Two extreme examples: one pint of milk produces 400 calories; one cup of tea without milk or sugar, no calories.

Starch-reduced rolls help to reduce calories, but they are not sufficient to use as an alternative to wholemeal bread. By using a calorie chart in conjunction with the diet that follows one can enjoy attractive meals without sacrificing any vitamins or nutrients. The chart shows butter produces 100 calories for two individual pats. The average consumption is six pats a day, or 300 calories. To strike a balance between personal taste and calorie content, check each item against the chart figure.

An approximate guide is 2,000 calories a day while

slimming. The average housewife, performing her normal duties, could manage on less. The essential factor is the intake of calories measured in accordance with bodily exercise, bearing in mind the high calorific content of popular foods and drinks. The following for instance, are all extremely high in calories; bacon; roast beef; rich fruit cake; fried egg; ice-cream; scotch egg; chocolate malted milk. A daily walk of four to five miles is regarded as the minimum for exercise.

Suggested slimming diet:

> the juice of two lemons, or one glass of unsweetened grape juice first thing every morning; raw salads, including celery and cabbage; freshly cooked vegetables; fresh fruit, but not bananas; clear soups; crispbreads; plain cracker biscuits; cereals, including breakfast cereals; bran packet mixtures; low-fat cheese; cheese spreads; eggs, not fried in fat; whole-grain foods; nuts; vegetable juices; vegetable oils.

Avoid:

> white bread; pastry; butter and products containing butter; salt and spicy mixtures; alcohol, especially spirits; vinegar; mayonnaise; cakes; chocolates; potatoes; peas; broad beans.

It is important to remember that no alcohol is the golden rule for slimmers. Alcohol is oxidized very quickly, which therefore allows fat previously consumed to remain in the body while the alcohol is burned up. Obesity is not merely a serious disease. It throws an added strain on the heart, with dire consequences for the elderly, if they attempt any sudden exertion beyond normal routine.

The simplest method of slimming is cutting down one's food by 15%, enjoying carefully balanced meals, but reducing the number of calories. Briefly, slimming is a combination of diet, exercise and willpower. There is no easy way! The late Mahatma Gandhi, whose ribs could be counted from a distance of twenty yards, enjoyed radiant good health. His amazing vitality, at the age of seventy-five, caused consternation among those flabby Englishmen whom he walked round the campus. They couldn't keep up with his pace, and they were thirty years younger! Gandhi, an expert on nutrition, lived sparingly on health foods—*that* is the secret of abounding vitality and the royal road to natural slimness.

*Chapter 4*

# SYMPTOMS OF INDIGESTION AND CONSTIPATION

NO ONE DIES from indigestion. They die from neglecting the result of this extremely common malady. Nature heals through its function of growth and repair. The essential condition is to remove the cause of disease and ensure its permanent removal. Despite those wonderful 'cures' for indigestion constantly advertised by the media, it remains a very common and painful ailment. Probably 40% of the adult population suffer to some extent. It is only a matter of degree.

Briefly, digestion is the process of combustion between food, oxygen and water; then the food is broken up into particles and the end product absorbed into the blood. Finally it produces energy and good health—if it is the right food! If the food is essentially incorrect, then it necessitates the use of remedies. That illustrates the importance of correct nutrition, the main factor that ensures normal growth in living cells—the *right* food.

Nervous tension upsets the digestive function and unless treated promptly can lead to other ailments as outlined in Chapter 10. Also, faulty posture causes sagging of the abdomen, e.g. slumped over a steering wheel or desk, which contributes to digestive disorders through pressure on the stomach. Following a summary of the common causes of indigestion, I have listed certain effective remedies, including an exceptionally pleasant one.

Among the fundamental causes are bad eating habits, eating too fast, too much at one meal, failing to masticate sufficiently, reading while eating and failing to rest after a heavy meal; also the wrong combination of foods and flooding the stomach with liquids at extreme temperatures. Sufferers are often aware of the cause of their indigestion. As it causes discomfort without actual pain, they are content to abuse their stomach over the years.

When at last the lining of the stomach and the intestines protests, and ulcers and tumours form, then, of course, it's the doctor's job to cure them in a few days! Americans are high on the list of sufferers because their meals frequently start with iced water which chills the digestive juices. At the other extreme, their hot chili mixtures inflict further punishment on an overworked stomach. Pain in the stomach should never be ignored; for chronic cases, apply a hot-water bottle and send for a doctor.

Temporary attacks of indigestion caused by foods which the body refuses to digest, tend to pass off quickly if no food is taken within twenty-four hours. Some easily digested foods are: milk; eggs (not hard-boiled); chicken; turkey; plaice; haddock; lemon soles; porridge; yoghurt; milk puddings; low-fat cheese; ripe fruit; cereals. *Not* easily digested are: pork; beef; liver; salmon; pastry; veal; cheese nuts; fried meat; mackerel; vegetables. Vitamin B1 is recommended for the normal tone and functioning



ç

of the digestive tract (stocked in all health shops).

Rich, fatty foods need five hours to digest. During that time no 'nibbling' is the golden rule and no liquids except water and fruit juice. Children's indigestion is often caused by drinking milk straight from the fridge, when their bodies are hot and perspiring. Gulping scalding hot tea is another bad habit to be deprecated in children. Liquids at extreme temperatures act as irritants to the muscosul lining of the stomach, especially when taken between meals, or after violent exercise.

Indigestion is painless at first onset, but sooner or later the twinges are felt, and that means a visit to the surgery. Or, the chemist supplies an antacid remedy, or an analgesic tablet relieves the pain, but fails to remove the cause. Sufferers continue their complacent mode of living, if 'living' is the correct word. Pitiable existence is more suitable, caused by refusing to change their haphazard diet and bad habits. To prevent indigestion means obeying the first law of nutrition—a balanced diet, eaten by slow mastication.

A balanced diet contains all the carbo-hydrates, proteins and fats, also the essential minerals and vitamins to maintain health. Persons with any stomach disorder should not take acids, fats, sugar or salt. In the event of a suspected ulcer, pain or discomfort in the abdomen, change to a strict milk diet until a doctor has been consulted. Freshly chopped parsley sprinkled on food is an aid to digestion. Peppermint cordial, either homemade or any popular brand helps the digestion.

Crystallized ginger, immediately following a meal is beneficial, but make sure it is genuine ginger and not coloured and flavoured confectionery. Slippery Elm Food is a nutritious mid-morning or bedtime beverage, which can be retained by the stomach when other foods are unacceptable. A furred tongue in the morning is a symptom of a stomach disorder and a herbal laxative is indicated. The fur should be removed with a plastic spoon before liquids wash it into the stomach.

A word of warning concerning the practice of cutting up dried apricots, peaches, pears etc. to give a muisli flavour to the breakfast cereal. This causes stomach trouble because evaporated fruits swell enormously when they meet liquids. Mothers are specially requested to note this mixture causes indigestion and constipation. Dried prunes need twelve hours soaking in water, apricots, peaches and apple-rings twenty-four hours and pears thirty-six, before they become digestible. Raisins, sultanas and chopped nuts provide added vitamins and are ideal for making muisli.

The cheapest remedy for indigestion and flatulency is a glass of hot water. For immediate relief, Heath and Heather's Indigestion and Flatulency tablets available in health shops. Another useful remedy is Robinson's Indikura Mixture, which keeps the digestive tract clean and healthy, and gently stimulates the muscles of the colon. It is also beneficial for constipation, biliousness, blood pressure and neuritis. Papaya Natural Enzyme tablets form an excellent aid to digestion; made from Papaya—'the health food of the tropics'.

The following Biochemic Tissue Salts are recommended for gastric disturbances, including dyspepsia and heartburn. These tiny tablets are readily assimilated and absorbed into the countless living cells of the human system. Ferr.Phos. for gastritis with swelling and tenderness of the stomach. Kali.Phos. for nervous indigestion and stomach-ache after fright or excitement. Kali. Mur. for indigestion or nausea after eating fatty foods. Nat.Phos. for symptoms of acidity and irritable disposition. These tablets do not conflict with other medicines.

Persons susceptible to indigestion should avoid having acid fruits and bread in the same meal. They tend to cause fermentation in the stomach, which in turn causes flatulency. Healthcrafts offer three popular aids. Each performs a special function to assist the digestive organs: Bio-flora, Florus, Enzgest, all highly recommended. My last indigestion remedy is that delicious liqueur Kummel—a tincture of cumin and coriander and made with brandy. What a marvellous excuse for a lovely drink!

We move on to consider the symptoms of constipation, which are often neglected because there is no acute pain in the first phase. Sufferers are inclined to regard constipation in the same category as colds and dandruff, something that merely brings temporary discomfort. That is a dangerous conception of this ailment. Constipation can lead to *many* forms of disease. Poisons continually being absorbed into the system by a breakdown of natural elimination, cause a variety of physical symptoms, and the mental effects are an unknown quantity.

To maintain regularity and to prevent constipation, Linusit Gold—nature's Linseed food is my first choice. Sprinkle on breakfast cereals, or it could be used in many other dishes. Prewett's Honey Bran provides the roughage that is so helpful for constipation sufferers. It keeps one 'regular'. The special diet for constipation is included in Chapter 12 and it also contains a grim warning from the late Sir W. Arbuthnot Lane, the eminent surgeon and consultant of his day.

Potter's Lion cleansing herbs (taken dry) are a popular laxative with no purgative or chemical additives. Half a teaspoonful is sufficient, washed down with milk or water. Lusty's Herbalene is another herbal laxative that needs no preparation and is suitable for children and adults. For children's constipation a gentle stomach massage is helpful. Massage clockwise, following the direction of the large intestine. Children often enjoy prunes for breakfast. Encourage them to drink the juice. Also, bottled prune juice is available in health shops.

Senna tablets are stocked in most health stores and they have a more gentle action than senna pods. The juice of an orange or grapefruit before breakfast is a useful aperient. Inner Clean herbal laxative is an excellent remedy for occasional constipation; in addition it is now available in tablet form. There are several brands of glycerine suppositories which have a comfortable easy action, suitable therefore as an alternative to laxatives, or to suppressing the symptoms with drugs.

Bran is considered harmless as a stimulant to bowel action, but like all stimulents its use is followed by a compensatory reaction. Therefore, it is not recommended as an aid to better movement of the bowels. It has a large sale in health shops and superficially helps sufferers, but more bulk foods and roughage are preferable, plus more exercise to strengthen the abdominal muscles. However good the food, however well-balanced the diet, in the absence of sufficient muscular exercise, nutrition is impaired.

The power that built up the living organism of the human body provided every essential for its development and maintenance. When one understands about the body's resources for health, one wonders why anyone is sick. The gipsy walks beside his caravan, not to save the horse, but for the benefit of his health. There is an object lesson for sufferers from constipation and many other diseases. Don't rely on cathartics—exercise regularity and regularly exercise!

*Chapter 5*

# HEALTH FOODS, VITAMINS AND SEX

IT IS A PARADOX of nature that males suffer from nervous tension caused by over-indulgence in sex, while females suffer similarly from the opposite extreme—sexual abstinence. Although the sex urge is a third stronger in males and females need longer to arouse desire, invariably they derive more emotional and physical satisfaction from sex. Happy sexuality in married life depends on mutual sympathy and consideration for the other partner's feelings, as distinct from self-gratification.

In our modern environment, health foods and vitamins are essential to enjoy the full benefit of harmonious sex relations between couples of all ages. The basic health foods—meat, fish, cheese and eggs are high in protein; the body's repair material, therefore, renders valuable assistance towards buoyant good health. Also they contain fats, the concentrated form of nourishment with more than twice the fuel value of carbohydrates or proteins, weight for weight.

Sound nutrition is necessary for true affection and fidelity to flourish in the intimacy of connubial bliss, especially in middle-aged or elderly people. Sexual excess cannot always be restrained, but the correct food and vitamins help to restore the drain on the nervous system. After the age of fifty sexual vigour begins to lessen and intercourse becomes a different affair from the driving passion and exuberance of youth.

With infinite wisdom nature has arranged that lasting happiness can be acquired by mutual respect and the sympathetic approach to sex by both partners. In addition, honesty and frankness remove obstacles to a happy and contented sex relationship. Males are particularly warned against over-indulgence, which insidiously develops a cynical and selfish attitude to the opposite sex.

Correct nutrition helps promote satisfactory sex relations, as indeed it affects all other bodily functions. When there are nutritional defects sexual desire is reduced, but returns when a correct diet stimulates the upward trend in good health. The high incidence of impotency in males and frigidity in females, indicates that the popular food of the average adult is insufficient to sustain normal sex relations. Nutrition profoundly affects mental and physical health; also it influences resistance to fatigue and relieves congestion.

Vitamins and mineral supplements, although good in themselves, will not restore libido failure. They are, however, necessary for the regulation of the body processes. They function in harmony with sound nutrition to release the healing power of the body, thereby restoring good health. Nature has her own built-in curative action and inevitably hits back if abused. In non-medical terms sexual function depends on a healthy nervous system, nourished by sound nutrition and free from emotional disturbance.

The value of vitamins is illustrated by the effect of sunshine on Eskimo women. Owing to the absence of Vitamin K during the dark winter months they cannot conceive. When summer returns the sunshine containing Vitamin K enters their bodies and happily they can conceive. The essential minerals to promote good health are; calcium, phosphorus, iron, iodine and magnesium. Dolomite tablets are an economical method of taking calcium and magnesium in the right proportions. Kelp tablets, containing iodine are available in most health shops.

Vitamins are necessary for normal growth and the main functions of the body. It is impossible to maintain good health vitality and vigour without them. According to feminine beauty experts women need Vitamin A to maintain their youthful appeal and glamour. This fat-soluble vitamin is retained in the body, therefore must be used with discretion to avoid toxic side-effects. Available in tablet or capsule form, or found in milk, butter, eggs, liver, tomatoes, carrots and fish liver oils.

The Vitamin B complex controls the metabolism of fats, carbohydrates and proteins in the body. It is destroyed by some methods of food processing, so a daily supplement is necessary to maintain peak vitality. The B complex contains vitamins B1, B2, B6, and B12. Two capsules per day provide sufficient requirements. B12 is recommended for preventing anaemia and also for improving health and energy in older people. Vitamin B1 (thiamine) improves digestive function, retarded growth and nerve disorders.

Vitamin C is used extensively to prevent colds, dental trouble, etc. It is a water-soluble vitamin that the body cannot store, therefore most people need a fresh supply daily. It is found in the majority of raw fruits, especially oranges, lemons, tomatoes, melons and blackcurrants. Preserving and cooking kill this essential vitamin, leaving vegetables in water too long soaks vitamin C away. Natrodale Acerola capsules combine two rich sources of vitamin C, rose hips and acerola cherries, an excellent supplement for all ages.

Vitamin D is the 'sunshine' vitamin that restores the vitality lost in the winter months. It is found in fish, liver oils and vegetable margarine (Sun-o-life or similar brands). Also, full-cream evaporated milk, although strictly speaking this is not a health food, it usually contains thirty-two international units of vitamin D per fluid ounce. Halibut Liver Oil capsules contain vitamins D and A.

Vitamin E is the general purpose vitamin used widely with good results by sufferers from many ailments, including depression, problems of fertility and abortions, circulation disorders and rheumatism. It is an essential dietry supplement necessary to maintain good health, available in capsules and tablets, wheat germ oil, wheat germ embryo and wheat flakes. For more information I recommend the book *Vitamin E for Peak Performance,* published by the Rodale Press, Berkhampstead, price 12½p at the time of writing.

Most people's diet is deficient in certain nutrients owing to their habit of eating refined and de-natured foods. Vitamins C, E and the B Complex are the popular supplements to counteract these deficiencies, especially for sedentary workers obliged to eat sandwich meals. Vitamin C is also recommended to help restore the deficiencies of the ageing process of the body, when used in conjunction with the essential minerals mentioned.

The products enumerated below gave every satisfaction to my customers, and include those I have used personally with good results. No doubt there are others equally effective on the market. These are selected remedies that work towards the elimination of the ailment—not the suppression of the symptoms with drugs. The 'change of life' tends to slow down sexual desire, but afterwards it usually returns bringing deeper appreciation of one's partner and more physical contentment.

Gev-e-Tabs are excellent for the over-forties. They contain eighty international units of vitamin E, plus all the B group of vitamins. Designed for mature men and women they offer more and better nutrition for their special needs. Also they contain calcium, phosphorus, magnesium and the virility mineral, zinc. The sex hormones in women control the monthly cycle and their functions slow down with the menopause. This causes the symptoms of ageing when supplements are necessary to help retain their physical attraction and robust health.

Pure Cut Ginseng herb is available in small packets in health stores. An effective tonic, valuable in preserving strength, vigour and vitality in men and women. Only minute quantities should be chewed at one time and then allowed to dissolve slowly in the mouth. For an infusion, steep in near-boiling water for 10 to 15 minutes and then drink, along with the chips. This popular Chinese herb can now also be obtained in tablet form. Sunflower seeds and pure honey are in great demand for increasing virility, and both provide enjoyable eating.

In the health food trade we frequently have enquiries for aphrodisiacs, foods or drugs that stimulate sexual desire. With certain persons these products may have that side-effect although unintentional, but that virtue is not claimed by the manufacturers. Melbrosia For Men are supplementary tablets containing 98% pollen. They are designed to counteract loss of virility and guaranteed free from drugs. They provide a safe insurance against nutritional deficiencies and the strain and stress of the rat race.

Melbrosia For Women help women keep their physical charms, and make them look and feel better. They dispel that tired, worn-out appearance that causes husbands to look around for more youthful companions. Celaton CH3 gives zest to life and strengthens heart, circulation and glands; it also alleviates anxieties and depression. It combats nervous tension and develops energy and vitality for men and women. By assisting deep and undisturbed sleep, these tablets are of special benefit to nervous or neurotic subjects.

Cernelle Beltux tablets contain multivitamins plus pollen. They are invaluable for nervous exhaustion and for restoring vitality to the over-forties. A great tonic that gives middle-aged people a new zest for living.

Cernelle Special Pollen Tablets are quick acting and invigorating. They restore virility and youthful exuberance to middle-aged and elderly people. Non-allergic and without any deleterious side-effects, they are a safe, reliable pick-me-up. The five supplements quoted above are sold only for the purpose printed on the package, or on the leaflet inside. They are not intended for any other purpose or effect.

Excessive sexual intercourse inevitably leads to a marked deterioration in physical health. The long term result is impaired vitality, loss of confidence and nervous irritability that affects the partners. Happiness in life means giving and receiving equally; one-sided giving is inconsistent with unity and tends to destroy affection. God's greatest gift to man is a marvellous self-healing body, that hates man's blundering efforts to stimulate or improve it.

*Chapter 6*

# COUGHS AND COLDS

WHAT IS A common cold? According to medical opinion it is a short illness in which the local disorder is in the respiratory tract and where mainly nasal symptoms prevail. Millions of pounds have been spent by researchers in a vain effort to find a cure for the cold, but so far without success. Common sense indicates the urgent need for prevention by any method available. But common sense is not fashionable in our drug-ridden sophisticated society. We are also informed a cold is caused by viruses, minute parasites that exist within the living cell.

Since there are over a hundred viruses that can cause a cold, it is vital to assist the body in its efforts to protect itself from these injurious viruses. The obvious method of prevention is to build up the body's resistance to the point where it becomes immunized to colds and other ailments. The body's general power of resistance is the deciding factor when bacteria 'invade' and viruses multiply, causing sickness in mind and body. One of the commonest causes of colds is undoubtedly faulty, or inferior nutrition.

For instance, sweets and rich foods tend to irritate the mucous membranes of the throat, rendering it susceptible to infection by viruses that can cause colds. Furthermore, sweets are apt to form excessive mucous in the system which provides a basis for colds and catarrh. Reason demands that we co-operate with the defences of the body if we are to enjoy permanent good health. Colds do not just happen. For every effect there is a cause and germs thrive best on weak, neglected bodies.

The principle of nature-cure is to build up a strong, robust body by the right food and environment, thus stimulating the body's own curative power. The injury that viruses can do depends on the condition of their host—your physical body. A well-balanced diet of protein, fats and carbohydrates is the essential 'weapon' to fight coughs and colds. Also, plenty of fresh air provides the body with essential oxygen, keeps the throat and nose clear and carries new life and health to every part of the body.

Nature-cure method is strongly opposed to suppressing a cold with aspirins, thereby delaying the elimination of toxic wastes from the body. The system steadily becomes more toxic and the last state is worse than the first. For quick relief I recommend Lanes P.P. tablets, the herbal 'aspirin'. They can be repeated in two hours if necessary without causing any side-effects or addiction. To relieve a stuffy cold, inhale a solution of two tablespoons of common salt in a medium-sized basin of hot water.

Garlic oil tablets or capsules have a remarkably good internal antiseptic action, and are highly recommended for preventing colds. Habitual sufferers should commence taking them in September to fortify their system against the inclement weather of the winter. The capsules are tasteless and odourless and have the advantage of being assimilated quickly into the system. Honey and apple cider vinegar mixed in equal proportions are excellent for building up bodily resistance to colds and coughs.

For a heavy cold, the primary remedy is complete rest and subsistance on a diet of vegetable juices and citrus fruits, gradually returning to full meals after the first three days. Deep breathing exercises started in the spring and continued right through summer will help to protect sufferers from coughs and colds. Orange and Halibut tablets are extremely good for the prevention and relief of coughs and colds. I must emphasize that these are a food supplement—not a medicine that relieves overnight.

For colds in the head a useful remedy is a menthol vapour rub, inserted into the nostrils and sniffed upwards. A small quantity can be melted in hot water and used as an inhalant. The old-fashioned remedy for a feverish cold is Tincture of Quinine, one teaspoonful in water twice a day. A useful head-cold remedy, especially for elderly people, is to soak the feet for ten minutes in water as hot as possible to which has been added 2 oz. mustard, first mixed with cold water.

Another practical remedy for a cold in the head is to mix 4 oz. honey, 4 oz. treacle, half a pint of vinegar, simmering for 15 minutes, then add about two teaspoonfuls of ipecacuanha wine. Thyme herb is useful to promote perspiration at the start of a cold, particularly fresh live herbs made into an infusion and drunk as hot as possible. Also, Yarrow is excellent for this purpose and is stocked in most health shops. When fresh herbs are not available use those contained in sealed jars. They are more expensive, but their medicinal properties are retained better in air-tight containers.

Let us take a closer look at that 'cold'. Are there any symptoms of influenza, measles (which start with a cold) catarrh, quinsy, laryngitis, dyspepsia, bronchitis? If a cold persists over three weeks, or any complications are suspected, then medical advise is necessary in order to prevent the cold developing into a serious disease. The most common mistake is to ignore a cold as being too trivial to bother about. A supercilious attitude is not always wise. It's better to be safe than sorry!

The biochemic remedy for a cold is Ferr. Phos. Tissue Salt No.4, and combination J is suggested for colds, coughs and catarrh and allied conditions. Biochemic remedies are not a 'cure-all', neither do they function with everyone, but speaking in general terms I have found them effective, providing sufferers were not taking drugs in the form of orthodox medicine. Huskiness caused by an irritating cough can be relieved by gargling with a solution of common salt—two teaspoonfuls to a tumbler of cold water. A cough should not be allowed to continue for more than three weeks. A neglected cough tends to cause influenza, bronchitis, laryngitis etc. especially if aggravated by excessive smoking. A pleasant-tasting quick relief for a cough is 'Balm of Gilead' cough mixture, available in health stores, and children love it. Also for quick relief use the juice of a large lemon and two tablespoons of glycerine, mixed with half a pound of clear honey. Take one teaspoonful three times daily on an empty stomach. If the phlegm is green consult a doctor—it is a very serious sympton.

Weleda Herb and Honey mixture is good for soothing the irritation of a troublesome cough. Crude black molasses is a beneficial expectorant for colds on the chest and a dry cough. It helps to expectorate the phlegm without straining the larynx or the membranes of the throat. An old gipsy remedy for colds is a handful of elder flowers and peppermint—make an infusion, strain off and drink as hot as possible. Also use Penny Royal herb for coughs and catarrh. The customary brew is, 1oz. to 1 pint of water.

There are seven Biochemic Tissue Salts recommended for coughs, according to their nature and consistency. They are Nos. 4, 5, 7, 8, 3, 2, 12. The staff in health shops are pleased to make sure customers have the right remedy for their disorders. Heath and Heather's cough and cold mixture is an effective herbal remedy that has proved successful. Benefit cough mixture is recommended for chest coughs and spasmodic coughing that refuses to clear up.

There is overwhelming evidence that vitamin C is effective for preventing colds, and new forms are arriving every month. The latest is Cherry-C-Chews from Natrodale, containing 100 mg of vitamin C in every tablet. Also available in health stores, super rose hip tablets and rose hip syrup for children. Because of its high vitamin C content, blackcurrant juice is used on a wide scale for preventing colds. Nature-cure advocates regard a cold as a natural healing process, a reaction of the body to excess mucous and toxins that are clogging the system.

The following nature-cure diet is not intended as a strict regimen, but as a guide to be extended to suit the individual:

> fish; cheese; eggs; lean meat in moderation; low-fat milk; yoghourt; vegetable margarine; salads; fresh fruit; fresh vegetables, especially onions and tomatoes; wheat germ with the breakfast cereal; wholemeal bread and cakes; olive oil or corn oil for cooking.

*Chapter 7*

# DIET AND SKIN AILMENTS

APART FROM parasitic infections the majority of skin ailments arise from faulty diet, therefore, our first concern is to correct the diet—the fundamental nature-cure remedy. When a parasitic infection is suspected it is wise to consult a doctor. In the meantime do not apply ointment which may, or may not, be beneficial, and could spread the disease. If the trouble does not respond to the following special diet, there may be an allergy to certain foods, which needs a closer study to discover the cause of the ailment. It is usually a delectable commodity of which the sufferer is very fond, but which builds up toxins in the blood stream.

Suggested diet to prevent skin ailments:

fresh salads, including watercress and young tender dandelion leaves when available; fresh fruit, except plums, damsons and rhubarb;
vegetable juices, all varieties;
cheese; low-fat cheese; but not processed;
eggs, lightly poached;
fish, but not shell-fish;
milk, but not starchy milk puddings;

lean meat in moderation;
wheat germ and wheat flakes;
real Scots porridge;
yoghourt;
wholemeal bread, not more than six slices a day;
clear vegetable soups;
verbama tea.

I discovered Vecon vegetable concentrate is a very effective remedy for skin ailments, although it is usually advertised and sold as a tonic. It contains 210 mg of iodine, plus vitamins A B and C, also niacin and iron. By curing a teenager's acne it gave me the clue to its therapeutic value for skin disorders. Subsequently it cleared up a chronic case of red rash accompanied by skin eruptions. The customer, a typical 'city gent' returned highly delighted with the result. In two weeks the rash had gone and the skin eruptions were healing beautifully—at a cost of one jar, 40p!

Crude black molasses is highly recommended for skin ailments. It is a blood purifier and has a high nutrient content. If the stomach is inclined to react against the pungency of molasses, the alternative is black treacle. Owing to their high vitamin C content, Aserola tablets are helpful for skin ailments, also they help maintain the body's resistance to any recurrence of the trouble. Brewer's Yeast in powder or tablet form is another popular remedy for skin disorders. Potter's Skin Clear tablets are a useful remedy for skin eruptions and their Skin Clear soap is soothing and refreshing.

When the discharges are clear and watery, Tissue Salt No.9 is recommended. Equally effective is combination

D which contains Kali.Mur., Calc. Sulph. and Silica. Peppermint tea, made from the popular tisanes is an effective remedy for skin troubles, especially when it is flavoured with honey. Garlic is a very effective remedy for skin ailments, and to avoid being anti-social, it is best taken in capsule form which leaves no unpleasant odour on the breath. Vitamin B1 is recommended for skin ailments and vitamin C is useful to furnish fresh oxygen to the skin tissue.

There are many herbal remedies having a basic medicinal value for several ailments. Their additional virtues are being discovered by discerning health food retailers who judge by results—having no axe to grind. The two most common skin ailments I encountered were dermatitis and eczema. Both were often caused by shock, and the former sometimes caused by handling metal over a long period. Both need medical diagnosis and special treatment, even if there are only a few spots and a rash. Shock is a very serious condition and skin eruptions can be symptoms of the body throwing off the effects of shock.

When shock strikes inwardly it tends to cause tumours, which need prompt medical attention and probably surgery. The diet already mentioned helps orthodox medicine to clear up skin ailments, but nature-cure remedies should not be taken at the same time. They do not compliment each other. The following incident illustrates the value of nutrition for skin ailments. A lady was suffering from eczema of the face, neck and chest. I gave her a list of the appropriate diet and three weeks later she returned to complain that she still had one red spot on her neck.

Skin irritations should not be dismissed lightly. They may have a deeper significance than appears on the surface. Some have an emotional cause which reacts on the bodily organs; anxiety, depression, mental stress, financial worries—the list is endless. Each individual should study his or her own symptons, bearing in mind the wide variety and number of skin ailments, ranging from acne to syphilis. The latter needs prompt medical attention and the former a radical change in dietary habits. The right food is not only essential for skin disorders, but it also enables the body to fight other ailments.

It is a slow process but the right diet gradually restores the body to glowing good health. Changing over to a health food diet can have its difficulties when catering for a family. However, it is well worthwhile when one considers that food is the best medicine, and a healthy body is nature's shield against all the diseases known to medical science. The science of nutrition means eating to maintain or improve health—not to satisfy hunger! It means balancing starchy foods with adequate quantities of fruit and vegetables, also the right fluids to assist digestion and the process of assimilation.

With a little ingenuity health diets can be made tempting and appetizing enough to satisfy all the family, including lusty growing children. Instead of cornflakes, try wheat-flakes sprinkled with a spoonful of raisins. There are many and varied menus which should include herrings, kippers, cod, halibut, lentils, soya beans, cheese and powdered skimmed milk. These are all rich in protein. The diet should also include salmon, which contains more iodine than cheese, eggs or vegetables. Dietary experts inform us that the most concentrated form of nutrition is the albumen of an egg, eaten raw.

Foods with a high carbohydrate content are; granulated sugar, jam, marmalade, chocolate powder, white bread, cracker-type biscuits, doughnuts, flour and cornflour. An abbreviated list that is merely intended as a guide for our purpose. Vitamin E is specially recommended for skin ailments and is included in the special diet in the form of wheat germ. There are several proprietary brands of stabilized wheat germ available and they contain additional vitamins essential for good health.

Here it would be appropriate to present a short list of external skin remedies, commencing with Hymosa Balm for minor skin ailments. Lane's Bolto foot creme is a useful remedy to relieve aching feet, also their athlete's foot lotion. To harden the soles of tender feet, try methylated spirit or surgical spirit. After-shave lotion is equally effective and has the advantage of a pleasant odour. To remove hard skin soak the feet in hot water to which has been added a handful of common soda. The dead skin can be scraped off with the thumb-nail.

Vitamin E Oil is especially beneficial for delicate eye areas—apply a few drops nightly. Vitamin E Creme is a very special cosmetic preparation saturated with 14,000 units of vitamin E—a cosmetic rather than a remedy. Simple Soap brand of toilet soap is recommended for sensitive skins and babies. A mild castile soap helps to prevent rough skin troubles, but used once a day is sufficient to maintain healthy facial skin. Vitamin B

Complex and Brewer's Yeast tablets, are the latest remedies for skin disorders, also they are helpful nerve nutrients.

Every skin eruption is evidence of the body throwing out various toxins and poisons created internally, hence drugs of a suppressive character have no lasting value. The body's power of healing is part of our inheritance, a gift from God dwelling within us, which indicates the standard of health He intended everyone to enjoy.

Your skin reflects your health and vitality.

*Chapter 8*

# SYMPTOMS OF ANAEMIA, ASTHMA AND BRONCHITIS

ANAEMIA IN simple terms means a condition in which there is insufficient haemoglobin in the blood—defined by the *Oxford Dictionary* as 'the oxygen-carrying pigment of red blood cells'. There are several forms and a wide variety of causes of anaemia, including the hereditary factor which is transferred through the genes. Furthermore complications arise because certain types of anaemia are identical to other ailments and only a blood test can diagnose the particular type and form. Therefore, we are obliged to discuss the symptoms in general terms, bearing in mind no two physical bodies are exactly alike, nor do they suffer the same allergies.

Tired eyes, shortness of breath, frequent pregnancies, pallor, general weariness, piles, excessive menstruation, are commonly accepted as symptoms or causes of anaemia. These are merely part of an extensive list, but they serve our purpose for this modest book. With the exception of those opinions expressed by certain eminent doctors, we make no claim to having any medical authority. The result of other conditions than those mentioned above is called secondary anaemia, and certain other kinds in which other organs are involved are called primary amaemia.

These divide into two main varieties—chlorosis and pernicious. The latter is a severe form of lack of blood, to which men are more subject than women, especially in the 50–65 age group. Chlorosis anaemia chiefly affects young girls from 14 to 25 years, and has many causes including defective development of the ovaries. Self-medication should not be attempted for this disease; put the patient to bed and notify the doctor. The symptoms of pernicious anaemia are difficult to discern at the first onset. The effect is so insidious that sufferers are unaware of it for some time.

The unhealthy pallor of the skin and a feeling of chronic physical weakness and debility are early signs. Then small haemorrhages appear under the skin, also vomiting and diarrhoea occur, accompanied by a variety of nervous symptoms. Not an ailment for self-medication, but if identified in the early stages the nature-cure diet would be beneficial—namely; fruit, cereals, vegetables, milk, eggs, fish and salads. No meat because of impaired digestion. but minced liver is sometimes given on a doctor's orders. Also vitamin B12 to supplement the above diet.

To return to simple anaemia which is the most common form and often caused through lack of iron in the diet, in addition to the diet stated above, I recommend two or three teaspoonfuls of black molasses on the breakfast cereal, and red meat is also necessary. The maximum amount of fresh air is essential. Miners and factory workers should make a habit of a routine walk every day. Because gipsies spend all their lives in the open air they do not suffer from any form of anaemia. Some doctors allow half a pint of guinness daily, while others forbid it—a discrepancy only doctors can explain!

A popular preventative is Froment and similar brands of health food which contain wheat germ, the richest natural source of vitamins B1 and B2. Vitamins B1 and B2 are the recommended vitamins for anaemia and are available in health shops in tablet or capsule form. Also helpful is the complex B group vitamin tablet as described in a previous chapter. Grapes and bottled grape juice are excellent for anaemia sufferers. Another helpful preventative is porter, the old fashioned bitter beer, now only obtainable in country districts.

B1 and B2 vitamins are found in citrus fruits, bananas, apples, milk, cheese, eggs, wheat germ, green leafy vegetables and whole-grain cereals. Iron is found in evaporated fruits, oatmeal, prunes, molasses, dried beans, eggs and split peas. Brewer's yeast in tablet or powder form is helpful because of its rich vitamin B content. Also available in health shops is a brewer's yeast and molasses tablet which combines two useful ingredients for combatting anaemia. A pleasant way to take iron is the new 'tonic wine with added iron', sold by chemists and off-licence stores.

Hysteria in young women is another symptom of anaemia, and is usually accompanied by copious weeping. The Biochemic Tissue Salt for anaemia is Calc. Phos., especially for anaemic children. Ferr. Phos. is particularly useful in the formation of red blood by bringing oxygen to the new blood cells. Use Nat. Mur.

when the blood is thin and watery, and accompanied by depression and frustration, and Nat. Phos. when an acid condition prevails. Another effective remedy for anaemia in women is the German elixir Floradix, stocked in most health shops. This contains iron in the form of a yeast-based dietary supplement, and therefore prevents nutritional deficiencies.

Liver plus tablets are highly recommended for this ailment. They contain 5mg of vitamin B12, plus enzymes, minerals and amino acids. Country folk use young thistle leaves for period troubles, chopped up fine and mixed with salad, after trimming off the prickles. Vitamin B12 is used extensively to control pernicious anaemia, but massive doses should not be taken except on a doctor's orders. Finally, I recommend Nutri-Time tablets which contain fourteen vitamins, including the essential B vitamins and ten minerals.

Let us take a closer look at asthma and bronchitis without fear or favour. Firstly, it is important to realize that the asthma sufferer is *not* struggling for breath. On the contrary he has too much breath; the trouble is caused by the spasmodic action of his exhalation system. He needs the assistance of a qualified naturopath who will develop his lungs by breathing exercises, and prescribe a nature-cure kind of diet. This has a cleansing effect on the system and he will benefit from the elimination of toxins.

Asthma is frequently caused by an allergy, known or unknown, the latter giving rise to more complicated symptoms. It is sometimes the result of respiratory troubles in infancy, bronchitis, whooping-cough etc. The symptoms are too many and variable to list here. We can only suggest safe remedies that have a general application to most forms of asthma. In case of a severe attack, especially if the patient is fighting for breath, medical aid is necessary without delay. Fasting is the nature-cure remedy, but it should only be undertaken under the direction of a qualified naturopath.

Children and teenagers are subject to periodic bouts of asthma caused by emotional upsets which in turn build up nervous tension. The upsets are minor incidents to adults, but they have an inward reaction to children, especially the highly-strung type, who are unconsciously trying to control their emotions. Mental stress—due to emotional causes, leads to physical tension, e.g. asthma and nervous debility. An allergy is often the cause, such as house-dust, eggs, milk, shellfish, animal hairs, pollen, moulds, aspirin etc. Nature-cure treatment aims at purifying the system of toxic waste, so providing immunity against further attacks.

Although there are several prepacked remedies on the market labelled for 'asthma and bronchitis', these ailments are not always present at the same time. A hard, dry cough and wheezy breathing tends to be a symptom of asthma, while pain in the lungs when inhaling is a symptom of bronchitis. Any acute pain in the chest could be a symptom of a serious nature and should receive prompt medical attention. Guesswork and assumptions are to be avoided at all costs. They add unnecessary suffering to the patient and delay treatment.

Asthma sufferers usually bottle up their troubles until they eventually become chronic worriers and slaves to habit. They should learn to cultivate the right approach to personal difficulties and problems. Logical analysis shows they divide into two distinct categories, those that can be mastered or solved and those beyond their control. The second can be dismissed and the first brought out into the open for examination in the cold light of reason. Place them according to their priority, then discuss them with a sympathetic friend and they begin to dissolve in the warmth of kindness and understanding.

Sufferers will find it difficult to cure their asthma unless they take the initial steps themselves. The road to good health is paved with self-discipline. There are no short cuts or miracle cures. I cured myself of bronchitis as a young man by practising 'athletic breathing'—simply take a deep breath and exhale slowly while holding in the abdomen. It develops strong chest muscles, powerful lungs and a strong diaphragm. For best results do it twenty times first thing every morning on an empty stomach. It is the finest preventative of pulmonary disorders, and its costs nothing!

For quick relief of bronchitis, take two or three drops of Friars Balsam on a teaspoonful of sugar, but it must *not* be given to children under four years old. During an acute spasm an occasional teaspoonful of brandy helps to relieve the congestion—again not for very young children. Deep systematic breathing prevents coughs, congestion, asthma and bronchitis. It means the maximum amount of oxygen flows into the lungs and oxygen is the basic essential to life. More valuable than food or water, oxygen is neglected because it is taken for granted. Shallow automatic breathing is more dangerous to chest ailments that the maligned English climate.

More oxygen means more energy, more vitality, more red cells in the blood and more poisonous carbon dioxide gas expelled from the system. Furthermore, deep systematic breathing relieves nervous tension, strengthens the nervous system and develops confidence and tranquillity. The appropriate Biochemic Tissue Salt for asthma is Kali. Phos. No. 6 which is suitable when the sufferer is in a low state of nervous depression. Half a teaspoonful of Friar's Balsam to a basin of hot water is an effective inhalant for bronchitis. The moist steam has a soothing effect on the bronchial tubes.

Garlic tablets and capsules relieve bronchitis and catarrh. Potter's Asthma and Bronchitic Mixture and their Asthma and Bronchitis herbs are both useful remedies, also Anti-Bron tablets for bronchitis. Heath and Heather's Bronchitis and Cough Mixture is recommended for difficult breathing and bronchial conditions in general. Cod Liver Oil capsules are good for bronchitis. They are a convenient method of taking cod liver oil without the oily flavour lingering in the mouth. Epsom Salts' baths are very relaxing and helpful for all chest ailments.

The basic diet consists of wholemeal bread, fresh salads and fruit, fish, eggs, low-fat cheese and yoghourt. Avoid starchy foods, white sugar, salt, fried foods, meat puddings, heavily seasoned mixtures, canned meats and chipped potatoes. If necessary supplement the above diet with vitamin D plus calcium tablets which contain vitamin C. Drink all liquids near body temperature; ice-cold milk from the fridge and scalding hot tea are strictly forbidden. Further exercises are good in moderation, especially if they have the ability to develop lung power. That is the important factor for pulmonary disorders.

For young people a daily cold bath is invigorating, but for the elderly a warm bath followed by a brisk rub-down. Then gently massage both legs from the ankles upwards, taking care not to rub downwards or press on any surface veins. Pure honey is good for chest troubles, and honey cappings are specially recommended for catarrh and respiratory ailments, but supplies are restricted by seasonal difficulties. Smoking cannot be condemned too strongly. It provides a constant irritant to asthma and bronchitis—especially if there is the legacy of a cough. These suggested remedies may fail to be effective if the sufferer is unable to break the habit.

My favourite asthma story concerns the wealthy business tycoon who spent thousands of pounds on treatment for his asthma. None of the doctors or high-priced consultants were able to cure him, so he retired in disgust and bought a small-holding in Somerset. This had an acre of rough ground. He dug this up by hand and this cured his asthma! The human body heals itself, given the opportunity and a natural environment. Merely give Mother Nature, who is a wise old lady, a chance to work in her own inestimable way.

*Chapter 9*

# HOUSEHOLD REMEDIES FOR COMMON AILMENTS

THESE REMEDIES have been tried and tested over the years, and include herbal remedies that are equally effective for many ailments. They have one feature in common, they are usually effective, except where an ailment is the result of, or the side-effect of a long-standing organic disorder. Drugs are mentioned in a few cases as first-aid treatment, they relieve pain and tide the patient over a difficult period. Their value with regard to the long-term interests of the patient is a matter of opinion. Angina is a classic example where drugs bring almost instant relief from pain, therefore it is wrong to deny their use because they conflict with nature-cure principles.

ACNE: drink Vecon vegetable concentrate and increase carbohydrates in the diet in place of protein and fats.

ABCESS: boil the leaves of red nettle and make an infusion. Or, wash the leaves and place on the abcess.

ANGINA: for almost instant relief, nitro-glycerin (or similar) tablets from a doctor; only supplied on prescription. Avoid; over-exertion, stress, frustration, rows and over-eating. Vitamin E is the best preventative, but should only be taken with a doctor's approval.

BED WETTING: Kali. Phos. Tissue Salt No.*6*

BOILS: Brewer's Yeast, either fresh, tablets or powder form. Heat a small bottle in boiling water and press the mouth of the bottle over the boil when it is 'ripe'. This will draw out the core without squeezing tender skin.

BRUISES: bathe the bruise in cold water. To bring out a bruise, bathe in half a pint of warm water to which has been added a teaspoonful of Tincture of Arnica.

BLADDER TROUBLES: Slippery Elm Food, also suitable for kindred ailments. Black molasses is very useful. Take a large teaspoonful dissolved in hot water and sipped after meals.

BACKACHE: P.P. tablets help alleviate neuralgic pains. Hot bath followed by a massage with Olbas Oil. If persistent consult the expert on the spine—the osteopath. Best preventative, vitamin E tablets or capsules.

BRONCHITIS: for quick relief (not young children) a teaspoonful of brandy. Half a teaspoonful of Friars Balsam to a basin of hot water is an effective inhalant. Garlic perls or tablets relieve bronchitis. Deep systematic breathing helps to prevent coughs and bronchitis.

CHILDREN'S BRONCHITIS: place the child in a hot bath and rub back and chest with camphorated oil, then roll in a warm blanket. The very young and the aged need special nursing for bronchitis.

COUGHS: the juice of a large lemon and two tablespoons of glycerin mixed with half a pound of clear honey. One teaspoonful three times a day before meals. Or, try Balm of Gilead Cough Mixture.

COLIC PAINS: can be relieved with a teaspoonful of ground ginger in a tumbler of water.

s: to relieve a stuffy cold, inhale a solution of two tablespoons of common salt in a medium-sized basin of hot water. For quick relief, P.P. tablets with a hot lemon drink. To prevent winter colds start taking garlic capsules in September.

CYSTITIS: Robinsons Patent Barley, it helps clear the kidneys. Drink two glasses before breakfast. To prevent cystitis becoming acute consult a doctor as early as possible. Avoid acid fruits and drinks.

CHAPPED HANDS: equal parts of granulated sugar and dripping, rubbed well into the hands.

CYST IN THE BREAST: an infusion of the herb Poke Root helps to control this disorder. Medical diagnosis necessary to ensure it's not cancerous.

CRAMP IN THE LEGS: massage the muscles firmly, stroking upwards from the ankle. Extend the legs and force them against the foot of the bed. Or, walk round the room in bare feet.

CATARRH: Olbas Oil helps to clear nasal and bronchial congestion. Also, relieves influenza, sinus troubles and hay fever. Full directions are enclosed in the packet.

CONSTIPATION: Ortisan Fruit Cubes are a gentle laxative that regulates the system. Potters' cleansing herbs have no chemical additives and need no preparation. The juice of an orange before breakfast is a useful aperient. Bran is the sovereign preventative.

DANDRUFF: wash the hair once a week in tepid water, using a nettle or rosemary shampoo. Include in the diet foods high in potassium, e.g. Brewer's Yeast, nuts, wheat germ, sunflower seeds. Best preventative, Vitamin K and Ginseng tablets.

DIARRHOEA: one tablespoon of arrowroot floa
'single' whisky for adults. For children, Tissue Salt Ferr. Phos. No.4. No food, only distilled water. If diarrhoea alternates with constipation it signifies a condition for prompt medical attention.

ECZEMA: hot Epsom Salts' baths. Drink Vecon vegetable concentrate. Vitamin B1 very helpful, and vitamin C helps furnish oxygen to the skin tissue. To relieve the itching and reduce inflammation, apply Morsep cod liver oil cream, obtainable from chemists. The correct diet is 60% carbohydrates, 20% protein and 20% fats.

EARACHE: for quick relief, insert a plug of cotton wool soaked in warm almond oil or olive oil. Fresh hops cut into small pieces and eaten raw. Or, an infusion of dried hops; drink a wine-glassful as required—children half the quantity.

EYE STRAIN: bathe the eyes with cold tea. To refresh tired eyes, place a piece of apple peel (rind outwards) over the eyes and keep in position all night with a bandage. Plenty of vitamin A, such as carrots, spinach, dates, apricots and watercress.

FLATULENCY: charcoal tablets or charcoal biscuits. Do *not* eat acid fruits and bread at the same meal. It causes fermentation that induces flatulency.

FALLING HAIR: massage olive oil lightly into the bald spot. Use a nettle or rosemary shampoo for growth and thickening. Deficient in potassium, therefore similar diet as for dandruff.

HALITOSIS: chew fresh parsley, or make an infusion of dried parsley. Stand four hours, then strain off the liquor and use as a mouth wash every two or three hours. Avoid strong tobacco, rich foods, spices and garlic.

HIGH BLOOD PRESSURE: Rutin tea, or if tablets are preferred, Rutivite. They relieve the symptoms and help all circulatory conditions, including hardening of the arteries. Best preventative, vitamin E tablets or capsules, taken ten minutes before meals.

HICCOUGHS: take a deep breath and hold it one minute, then exhale slowly. Or, sip a tumbler of cold water.

HEADACHE: to relieve tension, take P.P. tablets every two or three hours if necessary. Apply cold compresses to the forehead to reduce the over-distension of the arteries that cause tension. To prevent headaches, take vitamin B complex tablets.

IMPOTENCY: Keitafo Banlon pills, made from a blend of herbs concentrated thirty-one times. An effective tonic for health invigoration and genital functions. Also helpful for sexual frigidity, anaemia, and sterility.

IMPETIGO: dab the sores with B.P.C. absorbent cotton wool dipped in cider vinegar. Cleanse with olive oil and make sure to destroy the swabs. A highly contagious disease and sufferer's towels, sheets, etc. must be washed separately.

INFLUENZA: a teaspoonful of molasses dissolved in a glass of hot lemon helps relieve the pain and produce a good perspiration. For children Heath and Heathers Influenza Mixture. For adults, Tissue Salt Nat. Sulph, to be taken in alternation with Ferr. Phos. throughout the feverish stage. Nature-cure preventative, vitamin C tablets or capsules.

INSOMNIA: a hop pillow is an old country remedy. Calcium tablets that contain vitamins D and $B_6$ induce sleep without using drugs. After a hot bath, read light amusing literature, or watch comedy on television to relieve the tensions of the day.

LUMBAGO: for quick relief, lay the patient over a table and using an old fashioned flat iron as hot as bearable, iron over the pain through a sheet of brown kraft paper. Or, massage with wheat germ oil. Kelp tablets are helpful for lumbago and kindred ailments.

MENSTRUAL DISORDERS: Athera tablets are the popular nature-cure remedy, whether painful, profuse or prolonged periods. Floradix Elixir is excellent for this ailment, although not advertised for this purpose. In the event of hot flushes and depression medical advice should be sought as the patient needs assurance and sympathy.

MIGRAINE: Bidor tablets act on both the digestive and the nervous system in the prevention and treatment of migraine. They are not pain killers, but are manufactured specially for this ailment. To relax the muscles responsible for most migraine, get a friend to place a thumb and forefinger over the spine at the back of the neck, and massage with a rotary motion.

NEURALGIA: to relieve neuralgia pain, colds and chills take P.P. tablets. For acute neuralgia pains, usually caused by exposure, Tissue Salt Pherr. Phos. alternately with Mag. Phos. Orthodox treatment, paracetamol or codeine tablets.

NAUSEA: caused by pregnancy, make an infusion of gentian root—one tablespoon to a pint of water. To assist an easy birth, raspberry leaf tea, taken about a month before the expected date of birth.

OBESITY: Minima slimming tablets are highly recommended, available in health stores. Also Hofels Reducing Plan Formula S, a controlled programme that slims the figure and contributes towards good health.

PILES: Preparation H suppositories, are available in chemists and health shops. They contain a special wound healing ingredient made from Shark Liver oil. For itching piles, Germalene ointment. Bleeding piles need medical treatment to prevent loss of blood causing anaemia.

PROSTRATE TROUBLES: Hofels Protat has a marked revitalizing effect on the genito-urinary system. Herbal remedy, an infusion of parsley piert herb. Strain off the liquor and take a wine-glassful twice a day. Avoid, coffee, strong tea, vinegar, alcohol, fruit squash drinks, curries and salty biscuits.

SCIATICA: for quick relief P.P. tablets. To relieve those shooting pains, Pherr. Phos. Tissue Salt. Among several herbal remedies there are; comfrey, yarrow, ground ivy, and burdock. Do *not* apply pressure at the location of the pain. External rubbing does not affect the sciatic nerve. Bed treatment is often necessary, with a flat board under the mattress.

SORE THROAT OR LARYNGITIS: make an infusion of dried sage, stand for four hours, strain off liquor and gargle every three hours. Or, add 4 oz of red sage to a pint of vinegar and simmer for 1 ½ hours. Strain the liquor and when cool gargle twice daily. Sucking an ice cube often relieves the pain.

STYE: using an eye-bath, bathe the eye night and morning in a solution of salt water—one teaspoonful of salt to a pint of lukewarm water.

TOOTHACHE: if a cavity, soak a pad of cotton wool in oil of cloves and bite on it. Or, rub the oil on the gums. P.P. tablets relieve the pain and can be taken every three hours with safety. Orthodox treatment, aspirin tablets taken with water.

ULCERS IN THE MOUTH: Dinium tablets are highly recommended. Usually mouth ulcers heal in a few days especially with help of a bland diet. No salt, acid fruit, acid drinks, boiled sweets, or hot drinks.

VARICOSE VEINS: Stand in the bath, subject the veins to cold sprays of water, not too intense. Cirulinol, a German herbal supplement available in health shops is helpful. Vitamin E helps improve the circulation, also Ginseng tablets or capsules. Ginseng is not a specific remedy for any particular ailment, but a general strengthener of the body's self-healing power.

VARICOSE ULCERS: similar to the treatment for varicose veins, except do not spray with cold water. Instead bathe with a weak solution of Epsom Salts and hot water. Diet should include honey, fresh fruit, prunes and figs. If condition does not improve quickly consult a doctor.

WHOOPING COUGH: for quick relief, one good tablespoon of pure glycerin in a glass of hot milk. Gipsy remedy, cut an onion in half and rub the juice on the soles of the feet.

*Chapter 10*

# NERVOUS EXHAUSTION: THE INSIDIOUS DISEASE

NERVOUS EXHAUSTION is so common as to be fashionable. It creeps up on its victims slowly, relentlessly and unrecognized, until too late they collapse with a nervous breakdown. Let us turn the spotlight on those sinister causes with a view to alleviating the symptoms, without using drugs or shock treatment. With the exception of hereditary factors, nervous exhaustion could be described as the primary cause of the majority of nervous diseases.

Nerve disorders are becoming increasingly prevalent and to classify them under long-winded medical jargon adds to the confusion in the minds of laymen. Psychosomatic disorders is the current fashionable label, which implies diseases in which emotion plays an important part. Eczema and migraine are typical examples. While is it comforting to know one is suffering from a psychosomatic disorder rather than a nasty disease, it does not help the sufferer in the slightest degree.

The insidious nature of nervous exhaustion lulls sufferers into a false sense of well-being because there is no pain or apparent physical illness. They mistake energy for vitality, until the symptoms plainly indicate a nervous disorder. Lethargy, sallow skin, fidgety hands, depression, all betray a nervous disorder, or some degree of tension. Stomach disorders are a common result of nervous disorders; however the symptoms are frequently overlooked because there are no apparent signs of nervous tension. Furthermore, sufferers often resent any insinuation that they are suffering from a nervous disorder. Their familiar request; 'All I need is a tonic doctor', does not deceive the doctor. He encounters this attitude every day and treats the patient efficiently according to orthodox methods. The customary routine, nerve tranquillizers, sedatives, analgesics, etc. They give relief and the patient smiles with satisfaction if not contentment! But how long does this fool's paradise last?

Any subsequent emotional or physical upset (which may be trivial) and the symptoms return, or similar conditions, caused by the strain on a weakened nervous system. The seats in the surgery are beautifully polished, but is the patient cured? Bromides have the power of dulling the activity of the nervous system, while other drugs, such as strychnine, stimulate its activity. Therefore certain drugs stimulate while others depress. The challange of nature-cure treatment is that *neither* are necessary for the cure of disease.

Also the condition of the mind is caused by the condition of the body; both organs function together and both depend on correct nutrition for their nourishment and good health. To increase the supply of nervous energy without using artificial stimulants is the purpose and practice of nature-cure methods.

The basic features of nature-cure treatment are fasting under medical supervision, and the reformed balanced diet. They are essential to cleanse the system of poisonous toxins, thereby releasing the full recuperative power of the body. A diet to build up the health of the individual, as distinct from merely filling up the stomach and satisfying hunger. The purpose of the diet is to balance starchy foods with adequate quantities of fruit and vegetables in the right proportions and also to provide the right fluids to assist digestion and the process of assimilation. The role of food in health is that of daily furnishing the material for the digestive organs, but in disease food plays a more important role. If the food is deficient in any nutrient, the body suffers from vitamin deficiency and artificial stimulants impede recovery in the long term.

The symptoms of nervous exhaustion are numerous and variable. Certain patterns are familiar and others comparatively rare except to the medical profession. Owing to the limited space at our disposal we must prune the list to the most common symptoms: lassitude; neuralgia; chronic headaches; constant bickering; bodily tensions. These are all signs of nervous disorders. The golden rule is; 'Do not ignore or neglect any, including those that appear to be minor ailments.'

The automatic nervous system functions without our being aware of it. That is it functions to the extent of our limited ability. Beyond that level a feeling of frustration evolves which affects our emotions and our character. Our emotions depend on our vitality for their expression. Anxiety drains our vitality and leaves us a victim to numerous fears. To keep those fears in perspective is the art of relaxation and the pleasure of living, otherwise they tend to cause mental stress and nervous tension.

To prevent nervous exhaustion after a confinement three weeks rest is essential, especially if there have been any complications. Over-strained muscles quickly recover their elasticity, taut nerves relax slowly according to the standard of health of the individual. Brave smiles often camouflage an inner feeling of depression and deceive a sympathetic husband. However, watch out for the symptoms listed in paragraph three, also poor appetite and insomnia, both signs of nervous exhaustion. Unless diagnosed early on nervous tensions can be responsible for marital difficulties. They are the submerged rock upon which a marriage can founder.

Repression of affection is a cardinal crime that produces tensions in the mind and body and mental fatigue is the insidious enemy waiting to exploit discord. The compassionate approach of the old family doctor had more therapeutic value than mountains of drugs. Doctors appreciate the power of suggestion. The tragedy of modern medicine is that they haven't the time to practise it, because of the irksome conditions of the National Health Service. Psychology is an inferior substitute for warm-hearted friendliness and sympathy.

The two chief symptoms of nervous tension are, firstly, disturbances of sensation in the direction of feeling, or a perverted sensation such as hot flushes, tingling, etc. Secondly, it can entail partial or complete paralysis of muscles or limbs. Which type of symptom prevails depends on whether motor or sensory nerves are affected. For instance, facial neuralgia affects the main sensory nerve in the face (fifth nerve) and tends to be restricted to one side. The most common causes are exposure to draughts and decayed teeth.

Nature-cure methods aim at building up resistance to disease by treating the disturbed metabolism of the body. By providing better nutrition and a carefully balanced diet, these disturbances are avoided and the process of assimilation functions efficiently and naturally. Furthermore, the body needs essential vitamins at all times or its vitality is affected sooner or later. If these are not present in the daily food then vitamin supplements are necessary to maintain good health.

The wrong food, however adequate, will undermine the body's resistance to disease. This applies whether the disease has originated from emotional or physical causes; a glowing healthy body is the best insurance against disease from any quarter. An epidemic finds a waiting home in weak toxic-laden bodies. The law of nutrition cannot be broken or ignored with impunity. It is the foundation of good health. It creates the conditions which build up a harmonious environment.

Everyone's standard of health depends on their reaction to their environment, and on their ability to utilize their recuperative and healing powers. The common defensive attitude to nervous troubles; 'I'm not ill', is the main obstacle to a return to good health. It is mental exhaustion, the outward sign of inner conflicts and stress. A great deal of tenseness is due to having the wrong mental viewpoint. Sufferers should try to relax and to adapt themselves to nature's policy of non-resistance.

The following are three common nervous disorders.

INFLUENZA: has three distinct forms; nervous, respiratory and digestive. However, the suggested remedies and supplements that follow later are equally beneficial for every form of influenza. In addition to the familiar symptoms there often follows backache and neuralgia; also in chronic cases irregularity of the heart action. The common mistake is returning to work or school too quickly. The capacity for work (energy) is mistaken for restored vitality and a relapse is worse than the original disease.

INSOMNIA: a nervous disorder having a long list of causes with anxiety at the top of the list, followed by overwork and depression. Worrying about not sleeping causes the insomnia, which creates more worry–a vicious circle that must be broken, preferably by safe nature-cure methods. I recommend two calcium tablets in the morning, and two more in the evening, with a glass of warm milk. Get into bed, breathe deeply, stretch out the legs, close the eyes and turn the eyeballs up as far as possible.

NEURASTHENIA: can be caused by delayed shock, the result of an injury, or the accumulated effect of stress and fears. Sufferers have plenty of energy but are incapable of sustained exertion. A familiar weakness is feeling fresh in the early morning, but exertion brings on trembling and weariness. Also they fail to distinguish between essential and trifling matters. They are worried by groundless fears and anxieties, while lurking in the background is their real enemy–nervous exhaustion. When they learn to laugh at their own imaginary fears they have taken the first step towards recovery.

Laughter has a therapeutic value of its own, a treasure that cannot be measured or estimated by doctors. South Sea Islanders do not suffer with nervous exhaustion; their animated laughter and relaxed mode of living ensures them a high standard of vitality, the essence of good health. 'Nervousness' is generally the outward sign of a subconscious nervous disorder. The sufferer is subject to unrecognized fears that promote restlessness and apprehension. Unless these fears are brought into the open they destroy the efficiency of the individual and undermine his health.

Despite wide publicity concerning the harmful effect of cigarette smoking on health, it is a very common habit in all classes of our society. It may, or may not cause cancer, but it *definitely* promotes an increasing strain on the nervous system. Furthermore, to stop abruptly creates a chronic condition of nervous tension. It is better to switch to safe herbal cigarettes and gradually reduce the quantity. There is a new patent cigarette holder on the market that removes up to 85% of dangerous nicotine and tars.

Vitamins and mineral supplements although good in themselves, will not alleviate nervous exhaustion in a few days. They are essential for the regulation of the bodily processes. They function in harmony with sound nutrition to release the healing power of the body, thereby restoring good health. Nature has her own built-in curative action, which is directly opposed to sedation and artificial stimulants. She is often obliged to go to the extreme limit of restraining digestion, and refusing all foods before she can resume a balance of nerve force and continue the normal process of assimilation.

Vitamin B1 is the nerve nutrient recommended for nervous exhaustion, also vitamin B complex—the anti-stress factor that helps to build up healthy nerves and includes vitamin $B_{12}$. The essential mineral supplement is contained in its natural combination in Bonemeal tablets, a source of calcium and phosphorus. The following are popular safe herbal tranquillizers; Sunerven, Kalms and Quiet Life. For female nerve disorders especially the over-forties take Floradix Formula or Gev-e-Tabs. These are personal conclusions and are not intended to disparage competitive products.

The alternative to aspirin is Lane's P.P. tablets, the herbal remedy that alleviates nerve pains, are non-addictive and have no side-effets. Sufferers are reminded that herbal remedies take longer to show results than drugs. They function with nature at her pace. They have been in constant use for over 2,000 years and have proved their therapeutic value.

Another useful food supplement is lecithin in capsules or regular form—a food substance that is excellent for nervous and glandular disorders.

Here is the reformed diet mentioned in paragraph six, (it is not intended as a strict regimen, but as a guide to suit the individual): fish; eggs; lean meat; low-fat milk; yoghourt; honey; cereals; vegetable margarine; wheat germ; potatoes in their jackets; wholemeal bread; raw sugars. These health foods help everyone to withstand the strain and stress of modern living and to fortify the body against disease and degeneration. To eat health foods is to take the first step towards good health and the prevention of disease.

Dull monotony, frustration, loneliness, a boring job, all contribute in building up nervous fears and the insidious nature of these fears constitutes their danger. Unless the sufferer immediately becomes conscious of these hidden fears, they gradually bring about a state of tension that tends to be regarded as normality. Those early symptoms are danger signals. They must be brought to the surface however childish or unimportant they seem to the sufferer.

Disease does not just happen. All life is under the inexorable law of cause and effect. The human body needs the right care and attention and the reward is good health. If the system is clogged with drugs, or undermined with alcohol, then nature-cure treatment cannot succeed. The choice is drugs or nature-cure methods. There is no common basis and no compromise where one supplements the other. Nature does not tolerate negligence or abuse in the realm of healing. She responds with alacrity to the co-operation of a wise patient.

Many ailments that take a long time or refuse to heal, can be traced to nervous exhaustion as the fundamental cause. Only when tensions are relaxed can the body resume its normal functions, and poisonous toxins are then eliminated in a natural way. The inherent healing powers of the body take over and the return to health is a foregone conclusion. Nature-cure methods are unpopular because they demand self-discipline and the full co-operation of the sufferer, who is obliged to consider that results are not apparent overnight.

Nervous tension is one of many factors that, added to business strains and stresses make their contribution to the causation of a coronary, or a nervous breakdown. By cutting down self-generated pressure one can do more than planned, without feeling the constant frustration of expectant failure. Fretting over minor matters builds up stress to a danger point. In common parlance—take it easy! Adapt the daily routine to your own pace and live one day at a time. Cultivate a positive attitude—a negative attitude causes wrong impressions on the subconscious mind.

Diseases are not 'caught' as is commonly believed. They develop during a struggle between the disease-producing elements and the marvellous defence force of the body. To co-operate with the body's defences is to minimize the likelihood of poor health and disease. Sickness is caused by the body's failure to produce sufficient antibodies (nature's defenders) in a given time; therefore, the body succumbs to the attackers and becomes sick.

Environmental stress is one of many factors that can cause nervous tension. There are several alternatives that would prove beneficial, especially to sedentary workers. You could take up an outdoor hobby, for instance, like golf, fishing, or birdwatching, or you might change your employment or residence. It helps if you vary every day's routine and enjoy as much fresh air as possible. The lungs respond with good circulation to the correct fuel. The important factor for nerve sufferers is to get their minds off themselves. The wider their interests and outlook on life, the better for their health.

The insidious accumulative effect of nervous exhaustion destroys self-confidence, ruins careers, creates mental confusion and often means the difference between success and failure in anything undertaken. Sufferers try hard to live with it, but living is the wrong description. They condemn themselves to a 'vegetable' existence, when buoyant good health is within their grasp. It needs courage and stamina. Their attitude towards their illness causes the manner of its development, it is the basic factor that drives them on steadily to a nervous breakdown, or some degree of nervous tension. Their morbid moods and fears spoil their optimism and prevent them regaining good health. Optimism and nutrition are important factors that assist nature towards sound physical and mental health. Friends and relatives can help restore their confidence by adopting a sincere attitude of consideration and tolerance for their apparently aggressive manner. That merely reflects their inner frustrations and mental struggles. Their condition may have been caused by shock, after which the body often takes up to two years to recover normal function.

Sufferers feel lonely even in a crowd, although they long to be sociable and friendly. They are slaves to their own emotions and liable to endless mistakes and subjective fears. They need sympathy and understanding, especially as shyness is part and parcel of their ailment. 70% of mental disorders are improved when sufferers discover someone patient enough to listen to their symptoms. Their desperate need is *preventative* psychiatry, not as orthodox medical treatment, but as a general concern, like good nutrition, that can be practised by anyone. They need a well-balanced emotional regimen, as well as a balanced diet and the net result is vigorous good health.

*Chapter 11*

# TO AVOID A CORONARY

THE HEART IS capable of doubling its rate of contraction, and pumping out about double the volume of blood. This arterial blood pressure may increase by 30% to 40%, yet the heart stands the strain of this heavy load without any difficulty. But, two narrow arteries feed blood to the heart, and this is the weak spot where arteries may become blocked causing pain in the chest, followed all too often by total collapse.

Here fatty deposits built up insidiously over the years and if not promptly diagnosed the arteries may close up, causing that part of the heart to die. However, wise mother nature has a final ace to play; she causes other arteries to develop and take over some of the strain. The recuperative power of the body comes to the rescue giving the patient a fifty-fifty chance of survival.

The nature-cure method with its emphasis on correct nutrition is now part of the standard treatment to avoid a coronary. Its therapeutic value to reduce the cholesterol content of the blood is generally recognized, and used successfully in the professional field. In addition to the wrong foods and drink, nervous exhaustion, overwork, business strain, all make their contribution to the causation of a coronary. Although not necessarily in that order they add up to a formidable combination.

Tension is the normal reaction to life's difficulties, but it can build up to become a health risk that causes a coronary. Around middle-age the body gives out warning signals that it is foolish to ignore, or treat with disdainful indifference. Also, emotional upsets add their quota to the cause of stress and lead to muscular tension. We have now reached the stage doctors call an anxiety neurosis.

In this condition sufferers should consult a doctor, especially if there is breathlessness, or a pain in the chest, however slight or spasmodic. Nature-cure treatment demands a complete change of diet and habits, and will take longer to show results than orthodox medicines. However, sufferers will not be under sedation. Their symptoms will not be suppressed by drugs, although there still remains the possibility that they might have a coronary. What is important is, they have reduced the odds in their favour.

A brief word of warning: nature-cure remedies do not co-operate with orthodox medicines, especially drugs and barbiturates. The exceptions are Biochemic Tissue Salts which do not conflict with other medicines, but restore to the blood the constituents that are lacking. With advancing middle-age the blood flows slower, the arteries lose their elasticity narrowing the channel and conditions are ripe for a coronary.

Among the contributory factors, are asthma, obesity, rheumatism and the defective action of the endocrine glands. Despite some differences of opinion regarding the cause of a coronary, certain empirical facts are agreed by the majority of doctors. They condemn eating animal fats, being overweight, taking insufficient exercise, rich spicy foods and heavy cigarette smoking.

That a coronary is the mortal enemy of middle-aged, overweight people is an undeniable fact, and common symptoms should never be ignored even if the pain only lasted a few minutes. 'No one is tougher than their heart!' For the prevention of a coronary to those around the susceptible age of fifty, the following diet is recommended: cheese; skimmed milk; chicken and turkey; brown rice; fish cooked in vegetable oil; pasta but not in rich gravy; salads; vegetables and cereals.

Also, poly-unsaturated margarines, such as Sun-O-Life, which function with nature to maintain normal cholesterol levels in the arteries. In addition, pure vegetable fats are available in health shops. To supplement this rather monotonous diet, add Froment or Bemax which contain wheat germ the source of vitamins of the B and E group. Instead of white sugar use honey, it soothes the nerves and is easily assimilated.

Normal healthy persons having plenty of exercise may indulge in other foods in moderation, but watch out for the first sign of heart trouble—breathlessness. For a complete change of diet try the vegetarian foods in packets, they make delicious savouries, fritters, etc. The popular vitamins for the relief of stress, anxiety and increasing strain are the B group. These include the whole range of vitamin B complex, namely, $B_1$, $B_2$, $B_6$, and $B_{12}$.

The essential mineral to prevent a coronary is potassium, found in green leafy vegetables; it is also an ingredient of the Tissue Salts, Kali. Phos. and Kali. Sulph., and is recommended for dizziness, one of the early warning signals. Potassium is also an ingredient of crude black molasses and cider vinegar. The dosage of molasses is one teaspoon daily dissolved in hot water. Cider vinegar is best taken fifty-fifty with honey.

Garlic is extremely useful for reducing the cholesterol content of the blood; and garlic capsules help one to take garlic without leaving an unpleasant odour on the breath. Two capsules contain the equivalent of 50 grammes of garlic juice. Vitamin E's ability to promote the supply of oxygen all over the body helps to prevent a coronary and tends to relieve all circulation troubles. The latest anti-stress tablet is G.E.B. which contains ginseng, the great body rejuvenator, and vitamin B6 the 'nerve' vitamin.

The level of cholesterol rises when individuals face acute mental stress and falls when the crisis is over. Therefore, frequent emotional upsets tend to cause high blood pressure with its accumulative effect on the coronary arteries. The important factor is to balance the calories with the amount of daily exercise; to maintain the equilibrium between exercise, food and stress. Self discipline will avoid a coronary more effectively than medicine or medical treatment.

Around 2,500 calories a day would be sufficient for people around the sixty to seventy age group, more if they spend the day gardening or playing golf. Let us evaluate six popular foods that feature prominently in the mass food market. One adult portion of roast beef has

300 calories, ham has 200, a pint of milk 400, three slices of fried bacon 340, a third of a pint of ice-cream 205, and fruit cake 300 calories, making a total 1,745. The danger of eating these, or similar high protein foods twice daily becomes apparent.

To maintain normal blood pressure they must be balanced with low calorie carbohydrates, e.g. fruit, vegetables, low-fat cottage cheese, plain cracker biscuits, etc. High calorie foods hold a second threat to the heart—they are also too high in fat content. Here the question arises what amount of exercise is necessary to burn up those 2,500 calories. A four to five mile walk daily would be beneficial, using an even steady pace and an upright posture. Slouching causes tension and strain on the spine. Twenty minutes deep breathing, followed by bending and stretching exercises daily before breakfast, keeps the circulation in trim. Before starting a course of regular exercises a medical check-up is a wise precaution. There might be some degree of muscle imbalance of which the patient is unaware. It is quite common and needs *corrective* exercises under professional supervision.

Exercise enlarges the arteries allowing the blood to flow normally and ensures the heart receives adequate supplies, abdominal exercises help the circulation and digestive systems to function as nature intended, and the heart responds without strain or 'temper'. Health magazines advertise many suitable courses of exercise, but make sure of your doctor's approval, especially if there is any history of a rheumatic condition. The heart needs regular rhythmic exercise and a resting pulse of around 70 to 74 times a minute.

A coronary is not always fatal. Some people recover, but it is exceedingly painful and leaves the lurking shadow of a second attack. Generous mother nature usually gives about three months advance warning of a serious heart disorder.

That tense feeling in the head is one of nature's early warning signals that should not be disregarded. To practise prevention methods in the preservation of good health is not only following nature-cure principles — it's plain common-sense.

Vitamin E is now being used to prevent a coronary by many doctors, but also to help patients recover after the initial attack. Although doctors have different views on therapeutic value of vitamin E, there is general agreement of its effect on the metabolism of protein and fats. The most economical way of taking vitamin E is natural wheat germ which contains vitamins B and E. The naked truth is coronary thrombosis is *the* most dangerous killer in our midst.

To summarize:

A regular medical check-up after forty-five.
Correct diet to reduce cholesterol level in the blood.
The pain in the chest may not be indigestion!
Breathing exercises every morning.
Alcohol in strict moderation.
Plenty of walking, or a round of golf.
Reduce smoking to the minimum.
Remember obesity is an invitation to a coronary.
To avoid a coronary is to enjoy
buoyant good health into ripe old age.

*Chapter 12*

# CANCER, A DISEASE OF CIVILIZATION

'IN EVERY CASE I found the patient was suffering from chronic intestinal stasis (constipation) and that the infection of cancer was an indirect consequence of this condition. The physical signs of stasis are very constant and definite. The skin is sallow, fatless and inelastic. It is stained in the brown coloration regions, commencing in the back of the neck and the eyelids. I have found that in cancer of the breast nine women out of ten suffering from this disease were constipated.

'If they had been warned ten or fifteen years before, they would never have suffered from tumours or cancer of the breast. Cancer of the stomach unquestionably often begins in ulcer of the stomach, and that the consumption of irritating food, highly seasoned or spiced, may cause the origin of cancer to those susceptible. The principle thing to do with cancer is to prevent it, especially as apparently it can be prevented without overmuch difficulty.

'Chronic constipation is caused to a large extent by vitamin starvation, by the faulty food of civilisation, by conventions which cause us to delay and suppress the needs of our bodies, and lastly kinks in the bowels. Cancer in its early and curable stage, may give rise to no pain or illhealth; as cancer is caused by wrong living, the only true remedy is right living.' After all, prevention of cancer is the only certain remedy we have, while the cure by operation is to say the least, very problematical, very speculative and often disappointing.'

The aforementioned caustic opinion was expressed by Sir W. Arbuthnot Lane, Bart. C.B.M.S. etc. consulting surgeon of Guys Hospital, nearly fifty years ago. It is quoted from the book *Cancer* by J. Ellis Barke and appears here by kind permission of the publishers, John Murray of London. Those ominous words of warning went unheeded because the book was written by a layman, therefore viewed with that traditional barrier of snobbishness and prejudice that laymen writers encounter today. Fifty years later the estimated deaths in 1973 in the U.K. and America from cancer was 350,000!

Doctor Issel's success by using nature-cure methods confirms the eminent surgeon's opinion, but shortage of funds and staff caused the worthy doctor to close down his clinic which was doing such great work. In addition we have the book by Doctor G. Bicler M.D., *Food Is Your Best Medicine,* with many examples of cures by treatment along nature-cure lines. These are authentic case histories of remarkable cures without drugs or surgery. Cases drawn from the wide field of diseases as they happened—not restricted to the narrow confines of a particular ailment.

The great human tragedy is that nature-cure methods have been ignored by the majority of orthodox practitioners, and, inexplicably by medical science. Surely the science of nutrition is more important to mankind than scrutinizing microscopic slide germs! Medical science has made great strides in recent years in the early diagnosis and treatment of cancer. It is now usually cured, provided (and here is the crunch) it is identified in its early stages. Frequently diagnosis is made too late, because the patient felt no pain at the beginning, merely some discomfort which was not considered worthwhile bothering about.

Briefly, these are an abridged list of common signs that might imply a cancer. They are possibilities only and no cause for alarm. These signs may not have anything to do with cancer, but the earlier cancer is identified, the better the chance of a complete cure. They are: unfamiliar lumps or swellings; chronic stomach-ache accompanied by diarrhoea; unusual discharges; bladder disorders; sallow skin; unexplained loss of weight; lump in the breast; prostrate troubles. A professional diagnosis that is negative brings relief and reassurance. If positive, the disease can be cured at the onset.

Cancer is a disease of civilization and statistics show that it is virtually unknown among primitive peoples. Therefore its causation, to a certain extent, lies in the modern mode of living. Faulty diet, wrong environment, malnutrition, poor hygiene, alcohol, drugs, etc., all contribute to the development of cancer. These have the cumulative effect of building up toxins in the body; until these toxins are eliminated naturally, degenerate disease will continue to increase and multiply. Also, over-exposure to sunlight is one factor among many that can cause skin cancers—that lovely tan is a health risk!

Somewhere along the line of evolution man surrendered his hereditary skill to the 'gods' of academic knowledge. Prevention is surely better than cure, yet simple preventative remedies are ignored, while millions are spent seeking a micro-organism that may not exist! A few hundred pounds diverted to educational purposes, to extol the virtues of prevention is long overdue. The publicity campaign against smoking misses the target. It is not proved that smoking is the main cause of cancer—it aggravates it *after* it has formed.

The ponderous medical machine grinds relentlessly onwards. The gullible public generously fork out the money, but so far it has failed to produce results. Apparently cancer is neither infectious nor hereditary, therefore prompt action now would have a salutary effect on the rapid increase of the disease. Of thousands of drugs tested over the years few have proved to have any permanent value for curing cancer. Some are beneficial while others have harmful side-effects. Infection is not solely a question of the strength of the bacteria. It is also a matter of the condition of the host, your body.

The various poisons producing cancer lead as a rule to a cancer outbreak in about thirty years. Therefore it is obvious that cancer cannot be expected to attack the young. The cancer age usually begins around forty-five, but the age figure continues to fall as the disease increases rapidly each year. It is now finding younger victims. The age group thirty to thirty-five is not uncommon. This tendency could affect children in the near future—a probability that must be checked at all costs.

The old family doctors gave 90% of their patients a laxative as the initial bottle of medicine. Naturally it did them a power of good and they cheerfully paid up their guineas. Those wise physicians operated on the principle that a healthy body can be cured of most diseases—an unhealthy one presents numerous difficulties and problems. Constipation affects every organ. Vitality is undermined, mental efficiency is impaired and the joy goes out of living. Colic, the spasmodic pain in the abdomen, that often accompanies constipation, can be relieved by Mag.Phos.Tissue Salt, taken with a little hot water at regular intervals.

Here it would be timely and appropriate to present the nature-cure diet for constipation:

> bran; celery; raw carrots; raw onions; apples; figs; prunes; green vegetables; wholemeal bread; plenty of fluids.

Do not soak the vegetables in water. They tend to lose their vitamin content and a proportion of their minerals. To provide essential 'roughage', Weetabix or a similar whole wheat cereal which contains vitamins Niacin, B2 (Riboflavin) and B1 (Thiamine) and iron.

These vitamins are found in green leafy vegetables, whole grain cereals, citrus fruits, bananas, eggs, tomatoes and apples. For people who prefer their vitamins as supplements they are available in health shops in tablet form, or capsules for quick assimilation. Iron tonics and mixtures that contain iron, have a tendency to cause constipation. Therefore it is important to adjust one's diet in the spring, when most people take tonics, with or without knowing the iron content. Tonics sometimes induce an artificial sense of well-being. Therefore it is wise to avoid them unless they are prescribed by a doctor.

The golden rule for the average person is a balanced diet containing a high proportion of natural foods, with the accent on raw salads and lightly cooked green vegetables. To avoid constipation is to avoid chronic poisoning and vitamin starvation. That means avoiding cancer and many other diseases to which man is heir. When constipation is neglected dangerous toxins build up in their system and commence to putrify with unpleasant consequences. Nature reacts with a variety of symptoms, headaches, bad circulation, furred tongue, loss of appetite, flatulency, etc.

These are also caused by insufficient roughage in the food to stimulate the bowels, not enough exercise and excessive consumption of alcohol. Using patent medicines as purgatives is not recommended. They tend to create a reaction that leads to a return of constipated conditions. Nature-cure and orthodox medicine meet here on common ground. Both deplore purgatives and prefer the old fashioned remedy of the enema. Stubborn cases are relieved by injecting a pint of soapy water into the large bowel with an enema.

A spoonful of molasses or black treacle on the breakfast cereal is a mild natural evacuent. Plenty of water, fruit juices, a glass of light beer, are all useful, but too much alcohol is liable to cause obesity. Health shops stock a useful laxative breakfast cereal that contains bran flakes, honey and yeast. The juice of an orange or grapefruit before breakfast is a useful aperient. Grandmother's drastic remedy is half a dozen senna pods soaked in a pint of water overnight. Take a wine-glassful after meals.

Also available in most health stores is a brand of multiplex vitamin and mineral capsules, which are specially recommended to supplement the inadequacy of the average diet. They contain the eight vitamins and four minerals the body requires to maintain good health. The mental picture of waste food clogging the system must be faced, however unpleasant. It defies the natural process of elimination and nature replies with inexorable retribution. Bad or faulty drainage is criminal negligence and nature does not accept childish excuses. She hits back!

Cancer has many ugly facets and several forms of tumours to which the term malignant is applied, but many tumours are benign and easily dealt with by your doctor. It is the complacent and dilatory attitude that cannot be condemned too strongly, 'The swelling will go down next week' statement is not only lazy but useless and futile. If that swelling is a cancer it will *not* go down next week and the delay has enabled the growth to spread further into the body by the lymphatic vessels. The glands become affected by secondary growths if the original one is not speedily removed. It would serve no useful purpose enlarging on the malignancy of cancer here. It is mentioned briefly in order to illustrate and emphasize the extreme urgency of practical education in prevention. From the tabulated statistics I have lifted this figure. Deaths per million of the population from cancer in England and Wales in 1922, a paltry 1,229. Compare this figure with today's astronomical number and draw your own conclusion. Also the most advanced countries in which civilization has most highly developed, have by far the highest cancer mortality.

The terrifying increase in the mortality from cancer is an undisputed fact, an indictment against our eating habits and polluted environment. In the next fifty years will there be a repetition of the same dismal story? Will new men be recognized and given encouragement? Men with open minds and a new approach, who believe in prevention, in assisting nature to heal—not suppressing symptoms with drugs. We have too many societies studying cancer. We need more societies and individuals devoted to the *prevention* of cancer.

The science of nutrition cannot solve all the problems inherent in the prevention of cancer. However it has proved its value in recent years, certainly enough to justify further education and experiment in this field. A balanced diet, consisting of meat, fish, eggs, cheese etc. with 'starches' in the right proportions; a diet tailored to suit the individual, to build up health, as distinct from satisfying hunger, is the key. The maxim 'You are what you eat', applies to the prevention of all diseases. Cancerous cells do not 'invade' or flourish in robust, healthy bodies.

The cancerous cell will only grow in suitable soil and that soil is provided by the prolonged action of toxins in the system. Prevention is to lower our food intake, so that the former acids will not form again to pollute our bodies and lower our vitality. As disease is caused by rising acidosis, then chronic disease is a reaction to the same acid accumulation and only a complete reversal of our eating habits can possibly cure the disease. Good health is the result of self-restraint—there are no short cuts or 'wonder' drugs.

A reminder of the heart-cry of that eminent surgeon. 'If they had been warned ten or fifteen years before, they would never have suffered from tumours or cancer.' Well you have been warned. It now depends on you what benefits you derive from this warning! You can take steps now to prevent cancer. You can enjoy buoyant good health irrespective of your age. To become health-conscious is the first step towards good health and the prevention of disease. Your body heals itself within the framework of normal care and attention, and responds to correct nutrition with exuberant vitality.

If I have helped my readers along the road to good health, then I am content. It has been well worthwhile. This book has been a feat of memory. I have tried to avoid too many case histories although they would have filled the book. They are boring, except perhaps, to those with that particular ailment. It is said the best medical books are written by laymen. 'The onlooker sees most of the game.'

Finally, cancer is a disease of civilization. It is caused by bowel poisons, chemical poisons and faked food. Give nature a chance!

*Appendix:*
# THE TWELVE TISSUE-SALTS

| | *Principal Functions* | *Indications for use* |
|---|---|---|
| 1 | CALC. FLUOR.<br>Calcium Fluoride | *Maintains elasticity of tissues.* Impaired circulation, over-relaxed conditions, varicose veins, piles, deficient enamel of teeth. |
| 2 | CALC. PHOS.<br>Calcium Phosphate | *Constituent of bones, teeth, gastric juices.* Impaired digestion, teething troubles, chilblains, simple anaemia. |
| 3 | CALC. SULPH.<br>Calcium Sulphate | *Blood purifier.* Acne, pimples during adolescence, skin slow to heal, sore lips. |
| 4 | FERR. PHOS.<br>Iron Phosphate | *Oxygenates the blood stream. The Biochemic First-Aid.* Coughs, colds, chills, fevers, inflammation, congestion. |
| 5 | KALI. MUR.<br>Potassium Chloride | *Blood constituent and conditioner.* Coughs, colds, respiratory ailments, in alteration with Ferr. Phos. Children's feverish ailments. |

| | | |
|---|---|---|
| 6 | KALI. PHOS.<br><br>Potassium Phosphate | *Nerve nutrient.* Nervous exhaustion, nervous indigestion, nervous headaches. Stress due to worry or excitement. |
| 7 | KALI. SULPH.<br><br>Potassium Sulphate | *Oxygenates the tissue-cells.* Catarrh, skin eruptions with scaling or sticky exudation, falling hair, diseased nails. |
| 8 | MAG. PHOS.<br><br>Magnesium Phosphate | *Nerve Stabilizer and Antispasmodic.* Cramp, neuralgia, flatulence, spasmodic nerve pains. |
| 9 | NAT. MUR.<br><br>Sodium Chloride | *Water distributor.* Dryness or excessive moisture in any part of the body, watery colds, flow of tears, loss of smell or taste. |
| 10 | NAT. PHOS.<br><br>Sodium Phosphate | *Acid neutralizer.* Over-acidity of the blood, gastric disorders, heartburn, rheumatic tendency. |
| 11 | NAT. SULPH.<br><br>Sodium Sulphate | *Excess water eliminator.* Liverish symptoms, bilious attacks, flu, watery infiltrations. The 'liver' salt. |
| 12 | SILICA<br><br>Silicic Oxide | *Conditioner, cleanser, eliminator.* Impure blood, boils. Brittle nails, lack-lustre hair, in alteration with Kali. Sulph. |